The Art of Case Taking and Interrogation Including Other Treasure Works

By
Pierre Schmidt

B. Jain Publishers (P) Ltd.
USA — Europe — India

The Art of Case Taking and Interrogation Including Other Treasure Works

1st Edition: 2016
2nd Impression: 2017

Published by Kuldeep Jain for
B. JAIN PUBLISHERS (P) LTD.
B. Jain House, D-157, Sector-63,
NOIDA-201307, U.P. (INDIA)
Tel.: +91-120-4933333 • *Email:* info@bjain.com
Website: **www.bjain.com**

Printed in India

ISBN: 978-81-319-0244-8

BOOKS INCLUDED

- The Art of Case Taking
- The Art of Case Interrogation
- The Hidden Treasures of the Last Organon
- Defective Illnesses

PUBLISHER'S NOTE

Dr Pierre Schmidt is a renowned stalwart and has made a great contribution towards homoeopathy. Millions of pearls of wisdom are scattered over in the ocean of knowledge which were imparted by Dr Pierre Schmidt. This book is an attempt by B Jain to bring forth a few treasure works of Dr Schmidt under one bind making it easier for the homoeopathic world to access the teachings of a stalwart without much hassle.

The project could not be completed without the support and guidance of some of the leading practitioners of India. We would like to acknowledge our gratitude towards Dr. Navin Kumar Singh, Lecturer, Dept. of Repertory, D. N. De Homoeopathic Medical College and Hospital, Kolkata, West Bengal for providing us with the articles by Dr Schmidt. We would also like to thank Dr. Himanshu Sekhar Tiwary, Medical Officer, South Avenue CGHS Unit, Govt. of India for his guidance during the project and Dr KS Srinivasan for the translation of the article 'On Potency choice and homoeopathic potentisation'.

We present this work to homoeopathy with a hope that the teachings of a great doctor will be put to good use by the students and practitioners alike and will help in the development of classical homoeopathy in the long run.

Kuldeep Jain
C.E.O., B. Jain Publishers (P) Ltd.

CONTENTS

SECTION 5: TREASURE WORKS

Section 1: The Art of Case Taking

THE ART OF CASE TAKING

Today, I shall discuss the art of interrogation but first I shall mention one or two points about homoeopathic treatment.

The remedy you select may be of mineral or vegetable or animal origin or a nosode. If you are considering a mineral remedy, before giving a mineral remedy, please try to begin the treatment of your case always with a vegetable remedy. There is only one exception to this rule and that is *Lycopodium*. It is a vegetable remedy but please generally avoid beginning the treatment of a case with *Lycopodium*. With *Lycopodium* it is the experience of the old homoeopaths — it is so deep in action, like *Sulphur* and *Calcarea*, comprising the 3 big remedies of our materia medica — that when you begin with such a remedy you create a turmoil and you may have sometimes an aggravation that you do not wish, so sharp. And so, you have to be cautious not to begin with *Lycopodium* unless it is absolutely indicated. I make also an exception there, because all remedies in the materia medica have two phases — an acute phase and a chronic phase. We have an acute *Sulphur*, an acute *Lycopodium*, an acute *Arsenic* and so on. Sometimes, even a deep-acting remedy may be indicated for a short while in an inflammation or something of that kind but it has to be prescribed carefully. I remember a friend in Lyons who made two mistakes.

In the first case, the patient was a lady doctor who had a very high temperature. It was 43°C. She had at the same time a crisis of acute cholecystitis and pneumonia, and she was delirious and in a very bad state. She had received all kinds of remedies and at last the doctor had given her *Lycopodium*. In the acute phase with cholecystitis and lung trouble it is such a risk. At the moment when the patient is trying to help herself, to give the remedy so deep in action is dangerous, of course. The result was very quick — the delirium became worse, she could not recognise any one, and she was in such a bad state with high fever, trembling and sometimes with semi-convulsions that a priest was called in to give her benediction before she died. And at this time we were asked to see the lady. I go every month to Lyons which is some 200 miles from Geneva, to deliver lectures to 40 to 42 physicians there and this was one of my students in Lyons. So I said the only thing to do now is to antidote the *Lycopodium*. Of course, *Lycopodium* was her own drug but especially because it has an action on the liver, you know, it aggravated the case. She had terrible pains, she was shrieking, she was in a really bad state. Now she was extremely agitated, she was very red in the face, she did not know what she was saying. And with this high fever she was also very thirsty. So I thought the best thing is to give *Aconite* 10,000 first and then wait and see what we can do. Then she began to recover a little consciousness, she began to pray and she said to us: "Now I wish to pray with you" and she was always speaking of praying. So with this high fever, this agitation, this praying, it was typically *Stramonium*. So we gave a 10,000 of *Stramonium* two days after the *Aconite* and this moved us a little towards a better situation. But, when we came to see here after the *Stramonium*, she still had a very high fever because of the lung condition. It seems that the pain in the liver was a little better but she was extremely nervous and stood up with a 42°C fever to tell us: "Oh, I do not know why you are coming. I am extremely well. I have nothing, no trouble. I am cured. I thank you very much. You are very kind. But there is no need to come now," and so on, but she did not realise that she was so sick. This is typical indication, as you know, of *Arnica*. So we gave her *Arnica* 10,000. She rallied very beautifully and started bringing out some *Lycopodium* symptoms, probably she had had too much of *Lycopodium*. But by and by we could see she was better and after about two weeks she was again on her feet, cured. And now it is three years she is quite well. She was very pleased. It had been a mistake to give her *Lycopodium* at that moment.

In the second case, the son of this physician, who had given the *Lycopodium* had a sore throat, which began on the right side and went to the left, with a very dry mouth. He was very thirsty with a bloated stomach and he was asking for water all the time. He was, I do not know why, having irritation in the throat. The throat had one or two little white patches, and was very red with no ulceration, but he had terrible pain on swallowing. He could not swallow. There were some indications for *Lycopodium* and so his father gave him *Lycopodium*. But in such situations you should rarely begin treatment with *Lycopodium*. Please generally begin with something else. You can give *Aconite*, you can give *Bryonia*, *Belladonna*, *Pulsatilla*, any remedy in the vegetable kingdom except *Lycopodium*. So, he was growing worse, not better, and day after day the fever went up, he was not able to swallow a little even and he was emaciating? The father was anxious, the mother was worried and they were not at all pleased. So, I came and I looked at the case and I must say frankly that by taking the symptoms carefully I found that it was a plain case of *Lycopodium*. Now what to do? We waited three days and were watching the case. I thought of many things to do. I thought I would do what Hahnemann did for the rest of his life. There is a way to give remedy which is less harmful and less reaction-making — that is by inhalation. So, we gave *Lycopodium* but not the 200th which had been given already, but one inhalation of the 10,000th because he had had it already lower. So I gave him just one nice whiff, one little inhalation. But now, how do you apply the inhaling method? Hahnemann said, take one single globule of poppy seed size in a clean new bottle, not a washed bottle in which something else had been kept but a new fresh bottle that has never known any remedy, which is absolutely virginal. In this you put some drops of the potency in alcohol, and you hold this under the nose — one good inspiration there and you stop. You must realise that you are actually inundating the system with the medicinal energy. You are putting this on a surface of 81 square metres which is the total lung surface. In the evening the fever went down and the next day the boy was completely cured. His fever had been going on for 4 days, you know, and now in a very short time he was cured. This is an exception of an acute *Lycopodium* case. so I tell you, habitually, pay attention to *Lycopodium* and do not give it very easily. Yes, yes, Hahnemann said: "Give, if possible, an acute remedy, which is not Psoric, for acute cases and try to search first in the vegetable kingdom. Now, if you cannot get such a remedy, you may give a remedy like *Pulsatilla* or *Lachesis* from the plant or the animal kingdom, if necessary. But for the beginning you may use your *Aconite*, your *Belladonna*, your small remedies, we will call them small remedies, good remedies — very high in standing when they cure, they are then the kings of the situation — but still we call them small remedies, because their action is short. We do not risk any aggravation or engrafting something else on the system by repeating them. So that is why it is good to use them. Now, when you have an acute case begin with a remedy from the vegetable kingdom.

If this acute illness only came once in patient's life, it is quite alright, but if it is a recurrent disease — throat pain or headache or anything like that — the time to give that remedy is always right after the acute crisis. That is the time when the body had tried to throw the toxic stuff away and is the best time to let the remedy act properly. So that is why, when he has an acute case, the art of the physician lies in taking care only of the symptoms of the moment, of the acute symptoms that he has before him, not to take into consideration that the patient has had tuberculosis, or cancer — these are beside the acute things. Please think the situation is bursting out, it is like a flare-up. The symptoms are clear, the desires and aversions are typical. So give at this time, please, consideration only to the acute symptoms, to the symptoms of the patient at the moment. And this is not the time to take into consideration the chronic case — the tendency of the family, the mother, the father, anything else. It is only when you have no results that it shows you it is not a pure typical acute case but is an exacerbation of the chronic disease. And here we make a distinction. Between the chronic and acute, there is a bridge and in the middle of the bridge is what we call the exacerbation of the chronic disease which sometimes flares up. There you can give your remedy which first is the acute one, then comes or follows the chronic one. And an interesting thing is that all the remedies have acute and chronic phases and we must try to find what are the indications of the acute phase. Well, they will be very useful. Now so far about the question of acute remedies and chronic remedies.

In the art of interrogation, of course, the aim of the physician is to try to face five different kinds of questions which we must always have in mind very well. Of course, for the acute phases, please observe what you see and listen to what you hear. You must remember that Hahnemann said something very interesting in his Organon: "When you come either for acute or for chronic, but for acute especially, you have always a symptom, a symptom that you see yourself. As a physician, you examine the patient and you see what are the symptoms. But this is not sufficient. If the patient can talk, you must listen to the patient. But this also is not sufficient. Sometimes there are things the patients do not know or do not tell. And there are some things that the physician cannot know and cannot observe. If the patient has epileptic fits at night, how will you know this by looking at the patient; he won't know this himself! It is the mother, it is the father, it is rather someone of the family who can tell you. So you must know the symptoms of the patient, the symptoms you discover yourself or that he tells you and the symptoms that a family member or someone else observes and tells you either about his walk, his behaviour or his way of doing things etc. So we must have these kind of symptoms to start with.

Now in the *Organon*, Hahnemann was saying something interesting, that many people did not note something by which we recognise a disease — by the symptoms of three kinds. He says, recognise three kinds of symptoms: "Symptoms, signs and accidents." You know this *Organon* has been translated now for 175 years and yet nobody has ever understood what signs, symptoms and accidents mean. What is a sign? We know the signs of pregnancy. Yes, these are physiological signs. They are not symptoms because symptom refers to disease. There is the sign of respiration, for example which is a sign or manifestation of health. It is not at all a pathological sign. Now, in disease we have pathological signs. Hahnemann said very clearly, "You know *Opium* produces constipation and hard stools." Why did Hahnemann say so? You know Hahnemann never says something without reflecting very much. You know, constipation is something and hard stool is something else. Some people have inactivity of rectum and so have constipation even with soft stool. They are constipated in quality and quantity. So you must be very careful to know what is really meant by Hahnemann when he says, "*Opium* produces constipation following hard stool."

The sign is what we call the objective symptom while the symptom is subjective. Subjective symptoms are the symptoms described by the patient. An objective symptom is that which not only the patient can see but the physician can also see very well. But he cannot know if you have a headache — he cannot know if your pain is pricking, stitching, darting or stinging or whatever kind of pain it is. It is you who will tell him, so it is a subjective symptom. So this comes under the symptom. And what is an accident? Accident is a symptom which has nothing to do with a chronic miasm; it is something which comes from an external source. Suppose you burn your hand, it is an accident. It is not a symptom, it is not a sign, it is what you call an accident. It is not a disease that comes by the disturbance of the vital force, like whooping cough. So a burn, like a prick of a needle, which gives an infection or a sting from a busy bee or wasp is an accident, it comes from outside. Now, if you take some poison yourself this is an accident. It has nothing to do with the vital force. If you take away the cause, the thing goes away by itself. But you cannot take the cause away from a grief, you cannot take away easily something following indignation. This is something to do with the Vital Force and this is a subjective symptom. And you know that contrary to ordinary medicine, apart from the Psychiatrist, we are also very much interested in those mental symptoms — the psychosomatic aspects. For us they are very important, because they predicate the patient.

And for us when we take a case we must forget everything else. When the patient asks me, "Have you treated many cases of asthma before or this kind of skin disease before?" I say, "Good gracious! I hope I have not." Because I am not like some physicians who say, "The more I see a kind of disease, the more I am able to treat it." It is just the contrary in homoeopathy. We are like judges. "Because this one has stolen something is he guilty like that one?. May be that one is guilty, this one not". Therefore, everybody has his own case. We must study each case by itself. If somebody else has asthma and this one also has asthma the cause may be absolutely different and your task is to forget the twenty cases of this disease you had seen last week and to take this case as a new one. So when you have had many cases of disease, it is more difficult to take the new case because you will have to forget the cases that you have treated and not just copy and give the same remedy because it does not help. So what we must do in Homoeopathy is to be very careful. Every case by itself is a new case — you must forget everything before and after. But you know we are so prejudiced that when we see a case we think, may be it is *Pulsatilla* and you ask her, "Are you thirstless? Do you dislike fat and salt?"

And you know you are making the greatest mistake, that is to put into the mouth of the patient the answer because you like to find it is *Pulsatilla*.

I remember Dr Mable asking, "When you hear a tap open, do you feel a desire to urinate?" Of course, you would like to give *Lyssin* if the patient answers, "Yes". Again, he was asking the patient,, "Are you not sure that when you are near the river you feel like urinating?" You know in this way, by such questions, we are bringing out only very forced material. You must be absolutely independent and neutral in your questioning. But as our mind is generally prejudiced there is a way to get rid of it. I will tell you the secret. When you are taking the case of the patient and you see it is *Pulsatilla*, you write in the corner of your case paper, there, *Pulsatilla*. Now, after ten minutes, it is typically *Nux vomica*, so you put down *Nux vomica*. Then you see symptoms of *Arsenic*, you put down *Arsenic*. So you are astonished at the end of the questioning because you have twenty symptoms of these remedies that you remember. Therefore, your memory is very good. But in spite of being good, you cannot know fifteen hundred pages of the repertory. So first because we have put down the remedies, our mind is free, we are neutral and then after this, we begin to study the case with a certain consideration and according to Kent's and Hahnemann's method. Well, we will come to that later. But the main thing is first to take note of all your observations absolutely neutrally.

Now, Dr Gladwin as well as Dr Austin, who were my teachers, told me to divide the page into two parts.

To the left, you write all the pathological symptoms, the pathognomonic symptoms of the disease. The patient has tuberculosis, he is coughing, he is emaciating, he has sweat and so on. So your write down on one side, on the left side, everything that pertains to the diseases. For this you must know the disease, you must be a good allopath first. It is not a question of allopathy or homoeopathy, but it is a question of knowing your Medicine. So you write down very carefully all the symptoms on the right side which are the non-pathognomonic symptoms — the symptoms that are not habitually occurring in this disease. Let us say the patient is a tuberculosis patient and he has a desire for vinegar, I do not know what this desire has to do with tuberculosis. Or suppose this patient cannot tolerate fats. Why? For what reason this tuberculous patient who habitually likes fats very much is now averse to fats? We do not know. So these things you know are important which make you say, "Now, I have never seen a patient like that before." Let us take a patient who is paralysed, you touch the limb which is paralysed and you find it warm. Habitually, a paralysed member is cold. Now what is this funny thing? We have a description in every book, it is written that when you have a hemiplegia the paralysed side is colder than the other, but in this case it is not so — this is unusual! So in this way you are struck by these curious things and you just notice these symptoms which are peculiar, which you do not predicate with the name of the disease, they predicate the patient himself. There is the key of our success. You may not even know for what he is coming — for a rheumatism of the neck, a headache, or anything else. You may even forget disease condition when you prescribe the remedy on those non-pathogonomonic symptoms, funny symptoms. So please pay very much attention always to the non-pathognomonic symptoms. To understand this you must know your Medicine well because you must know what is the disease usually like — whether it is enteritis or cholera or anything else. You must know what are the symptoms of disease but, if you find something that has nothing to do with this disease, so that it predicates the patient, please value it. And you will make your best cures when you can find such symptoms.

I may say here that when a patient in any disease has still many non-pathognomonic symptoms (symptoms of himself) there is a hope of cure. But unfortunately in cases at the end and in many chronic diseases e.g. multiple sclerosis, there are almost no symptoms of the patient. You have only symptoms of the disease. All those individualising symptoms fade away. These cases then become difficult to cure. That is why I insist that you find the non-pathognomonic symptoms.

The first thing after having heard the patient is to allow him to tell all about the disease. Of course, I suppose you ask him first what are the things for which he is coming to consult you. Then you let him talk. If they talk too long, ask them to come again. They will always come and then when they are finished, you must not be pleased with it. You must ask, "What is more?" When he has ceased, still ask him, "Tell me more." So you must ask, you must express from them every detail, till they tell everything about their sickness, all they may know about their disease.

You may find sometimes, that after every symptom has been taken down, a lady patient coming back again with a long list of symptoms, giving again a different story. Otherwise, she will tell you that you have not had the time to listen to her, you were in a great hurry. So when I see it is a long case, I always say, "All right. Come along another time." So when they come three, four or five times they begin to feel that they have described their illness enough.

Now is the time to yourself begin the questioning. When they have finished telling their story, you begin to ask questions. Habitually, you can begin with the hereditary taints. It is interesting. You must know the patient's religion too. Why the religion? Because you know, for example, in our country Catholics have many fears — fear of the flames in the inferno (hell) which Protestants do not have. The Jewish have other kinds of fears. Then about the profession. It is interesting to know because our patients may have troubles because of their professions. So, of course, the first thing is to try to remove the cause. Then you must know how many children they have, if they are married or divorced, if they have any domestic troubles. So, when a lady has been divorced once or twice or a third time, you begin to see the symptoms which are very probably of the animal sphere, and it may be *Lachesis* or *Sepia* or something like that.

After you have asked the preliminary symptoms, come to the general symptoms. Of course, the general symptoms are such that everybody is supposed to be questioned about them. There you must know your repertory quite well. The first question is about the state of vital heat — excess or lack of it — which is very important. Then about the time of the twenty four hours when the patient feels worse, then about the climate, modifications, about the position, motion, about the air — snow air, mountain, seashore etc., about hot or cold water, about their clothing — if they like tight clothing or loose, about the question of woollen clothing, then about the food, what are the foods which make them worse, about the wounds, whether they clear up easily or they suppurate easily or bleed freely, etc. etc.

When you have asked about the general symptoms, you become a little more acquainted with your patient, he sees that you are interested in him. Then he is ready to give you some mental symptoms. Now, you have to judge if it is the time to go further. If you cannot ask mental symptoms, you can go on then to the symptoms of desires and aversion in food.

The attention to the method, how you ask your questions is very important, for example, if you ask the patient, "Do you like *Namak*[1], of course, the patient will tell you "yes" or "no". But first you must never put a question that they can answer by a yes or no. It is not so easy. In the translation that I have made of the original

1 "Namak"is a Hindi word for common salt

Organon 6th edition, is a series of question. (I made the translation because I found to my great astonishment that the man who had translated all the works of Hahnemann into French was an allopathic physician who never knew homoeopathy! Can you imagine? Nobody has ever found this out. Hahnemann has never recognised any translation as perfect. So you see when I saw many mistakes, in shades, in very fine shades, we found it necessary to bring out an edition where everything is written exactly as Hahnemann said). So Hahnemann has made the questionnaire which is a marvellous thing where it is impossible to answer the questions by a Yes or No. (But your English translation is not right at all. You cannot unfortunately rely on this translation. Hering who knew French, English and German was a keen student of Hahnemann and he has translated the *Organon*, 3rd edition. And we rely on this edition very much for many shades of meaning. He only translated the 3rd edition — not the 4th or 5th). And so about the questionnaire, there you will find two things in Hahnemann. These questions, they are fascinating. Not one question can you answer by a yes or no. You do not ask the patients, "Are you thirsty?" Because when you ask them, "Are you thirsty?", they think you are referring to soup or tea. Of course, you can drink tea without being thirsty for the pleasure of taking tea, but that is not relevant here. So there are patients who think that they drink soup when they are thirsty but that is wrong. Some others drink lots of water and think they are not thirsty because it is at the time of the meal. So you must be very cautious. "How much liquid do you need in a day?" or "What about thirst?"

They cannot say Yes or No. They must think. You cannot put questions like "Are you jealous?" So you have to put such sort of questions as taught by Hahnemann. You can copy them. They are very nice. Such are the questions that they must be answered by the patient without being able to say Yes or No in rely.

Another thing, Hahnemann has prepared 22 questions about diseases they will hide. The patient will not tell you the truth or will not tell you at all. And Hahnemann has described 22 very interesting different diagnoses and diseases or troubles that the patient hides. Either he hides something of his mind when there has been trouble about grief, or mortification or some wrong that the patient has committed that he will not tell you about. So you may know many interesting things by asking the questions that Hahnemann has put down. Of course, a homoeopath, besides his homoeopathy, is able sometimes to know things which the patients will not tell him. How is he able to do it? *First*, observation. *Second*, somebody has told him something before the patient came and therefore he knew something already. He must have good memory about it. *Third*, you have people who know graphology asking the patient to write something and you know many such things by knowing graphology. A good homoeopath should know graphology because it helps very much. Now nominology may help through the name of the patient. Every name is a vibration. The name that you are given when you are born is not something in the air. It is something that vibrates every time you are called, Paul or Samuel or something. This name has, in fact, a science about it. Besides this, there is numerology.

By the name and birth-date of the patient you can tell his character. At once, you know his tendency. You know if he is stubborn, very sensitive to beauty or form, or if he is a businessman etc. All these you know by the date of birth and if you have further a microscope you can look into his eyes and see by the form of his pupil what he is hiding.

For example, once a young girl about 18 years of age came complaining that she had been having constipation for six months. She had gone to many physicians and had tried many laxatives. Either there was no result or they gave such side-effects that she was sick many a time. Now, the question is, why was she constipated so much? She was going to the school and nothing was wrong. I looked into her eyes and the pupil which was supposed to be round was not round at all. In the 12 o'clock position was a sign of grief. She was suffering from grief but she would not tell — a silent grief? The ailment was possibly due to silent grief. May be it was *Ignatia* or *Nat. mur*. In a girl of 18, what can it be? It can only be a sweetheart and a sweetheart that she cannot tell her mother or father about, or is opposed by the father or the mother. So I said to the girl, "I think you have a grief connected with your sweetheart." She began to cry and the mother said, "Yes, that is so but she would not tell me earlier." This was the cause of the constipation. One dose of *Ignatia* and she was cured at once. Since that time there has been no trouble though I had to arrange with the parents and the daughter how to manage the situation so that it can be accepted.

So you see, you can get information even by looking into the eyes. Now, this was in the right eye. If it is in the left eye, it is not all grief. This is funny. Everybody is divided into two parts or two poles, the right one is the father's side, the left one is the mother's side. If it is in the left eye, it is a revengeful feeling, or rage inside, an angry feeling against somebody e.g. it could be a secretary whom the boss is criticising and fault-finding, so she comes every day already trembling and says all day she is constipated, because she is always under fear. So this is interesting — ailment from fright and silent or suppressed anger. In this case, what is the remedy? *Staphysagria* of course. What is the full name of *Staphysagria*? *Delphinum Staphysagria*. It is a plant. It can be rosy or blue. It has symptoms of indignation, angry feeling that you cannot express.

Sometimes you must be like a detective, you must make deduction. Once there was a lady who came to me. I was treating her husband and her mother and I was knowing that her family was absolutely harmonious. She liked her husband, she liked her children, she had a nice mother. She was not working in an office. She was at home. Now I thought to myself what can it be? It can be only one thing. It must be a lady, a maid, of course, perhaps putting the water into the flower vases so much that it fell onto the carpet a little or perhaps she put no milk in the tea, giving trouble all the time. Of course, I thought this lady cannot tell her husband because he will be annoyed. So she keeps it to herself. I said to her, "It is of course that lady who is making trouble for you, doing this and that." She said, "How do you know? It is exactly so." This is very curious and this is so when you see it in the left eye. Now, if you have a flattening at 6 o'clock (position) instead of at 12, it is something else, it means that the patient has flat feet. So you must give her something to put in her shoe. If the patient does not tell you this, it is very difficult to know. But by looking into the pupil only, you know this at once. Now, when you put a light into the pupil from sideways or so, the pupil at once contracts and a normal pupil contracts and remains contracted as long as there is light. Instead of this if you see the pupil always contracting and dilating, what is this? This is found in a vagosympathetic patient. Such patients have alternating troubles. They have alternated constipation and diarrhoea and their characteristic moods are always either up or down, like the pupil, always up and down, never at the centre.

So you see there are so many things to be learnt by looking at the pupil. I do not have the time to describe them all today. There are at least 10-12 diseases which can be diagnosed only by looking into the pupil[2]. Unfortunately, most of the books written on the subject are quite bad. The only reliable book is by Dr Sinabe in German.

Now, you have had a look at your patient and then you are beginning to note the general symptoms. You are beginning to take the symptoms of the stomach, the desires, the cravings etc. When a patient has a desire e.g. for salt, for *Namak* as I told you, it is not sufficient if he says, "Yes, I like salt". This is not a symptom. No! There are people who prefer adding salt *before* eating,

2. *This science is called Iris Diagnosis*

they add salt *before* tasting the food. This is a desire for salt. There are patients who cannot go the whole day long without a piece of sugar or chocolate or something sweet in their pocket because they love sweets. This is a desire, this is a craving. But when the patient says (in a dull unenthusiastic voice), "Yes, I like this, I like that", this is not a symptom. He must say that eagerly with force. As they speak, it must show on their faces — what they like and dislike. So you must be very careful about this and you will be helped by the way they answer. This cannot be weighed in writing. Only, you can underline (the symptom) once or twice if they really seem to be very typical.

By the way, it is no use asking the patients things that are not in the repertory, because that will not help you to find the remedy. If the patent likes almonds, for example, it is very nice but because it is not in the repertory, it is no use asking this question.

So there is salt, sugar or sweets, fats and sour things that you must absolutely know because they are in the repertory. Now, you also have butter, cheese, eggs, milk, meat etc., but funny to say, patients do not show so much craving for these, but the four things I mentioned first are very important. You know eggs are very important in our country because we eat many eggs, but there are only 3, 4 remedies given in the repertory. So in the repertory when there are only 3, 4 remedies, e.g. *Fer.*, *Calc. c.*, etc., we cannot go very far. Our remedies have not been proved enough to bring out all those cravings, so it is up to you to please try and add to our repertories by making provings and trying to find our new symptoms. So do not find fault with Hahnemann and others. Please try yourself to do better.

Now, we come to thirst. What about thirst, especially when there is fever? Suppose the patient says, "Oh, I never drink (water) when I have fever," this is interesting. If they are thirsty during fever, it is absolutely not interesting because everybody with fever is thirsty. But in a case when you expect people to be thirsty, if they are not, then it is very interesting. If they say, "Yes, when the weather is very hot, I drink much water," please remember that everybody does so. So please put this in the column of pathognomonic symptoms and take the other one "When it is very hot I never drink." This is a symptom you at once put down in black letters or gold letters. This is important.

Now, comes the question of sleep. You know in sleep we have been able to add different symptoms which you do not have in your repertory[3].

---

3. *In my repertory, I have put down the mental symptoms of Dr Gallivardin, a Frenchman who studied all his life only mental symptoms and cured many patients only by the mental symptom. It was his hobby to study mental symptoms and pick out the remedy only on the mental symptoms. No other symptoms — only mental symptoms! He cured so many cases, you cannot imagine. Patients were cured even without their knowing that they were taking the remedy because the remedy was given in the wine, even in the coffee and the milk and it worked beautifully. Of course, we say coffee antidotes the remedy but the coffee is in a crude state while the dynamised, spiritualised state of remedy is something quite different. But it acts still, even with coffee.*

   Among the symptoms I have added in my repertory is Adultery. We have remedies to induce a man to quit his mistress and come back to his wife. We have also remedies to wean away people who are drinking whether it is wine or beer. I have added all these in my repertory.

So the first thing that is interesting about the sleep is that many patients complain of sleeplessness. About sleeplessness, it is interesting to know which time he is sleepless. Now comes the kind of sleep, whether the sleep is heavy or if he sleeps like the cat, or the dog who hears with one half of the brain while the other half is sleeping. There are people who can tell the things that were spoken all the night though they were in a slumber, which is really not a sleep. It is not normal. This is not repose, this is not refreshing. Because it is the grace of God to have the sleep, this time when the body is free from the soul and is retiring and resting in the night. But nobody has been able to explain what is sleep. Nobody knows what it is. We have had many theories but nobody is satisfied with them. But anyway with homoeopathy, we can help this sleep.

Now, it is very important to know what you do while you sleep. Some people sleep with their eyes open. You may ask the patient but the patient does not know. It is the mother or the father who tells you, "Yes, the eyes are always open." In some others when they sleep, the saliva is running. Some others have jerks and give kicks around to the mother or to the husband. It may be twitching, it may be jerking, it may be shocks — you must make out the differences between them. It is not so easy.

What is interesting is while the patient sleeps he may be doing different things. He may be rolling his head this way or that. He may do funny things with the hands when he sleeps. He may sleep always with his feet crossed. The remedy, as everybody knows, is *Rhododendron*. Now there are patients who sleep in funny positions, square in the bed. Some others can sleep only on the left side, in spite of heart disease which is very interesting — only on the left side, with heart disease! This is just a symptom to which the homoeopath gives high consideration, because we will not expect somebody with palpitations to sleep better on the left side. And now some put their arms up above the head. Some people sleep like that, like Hitler. Now, when people sleep like that there is some trouble with the liver. Ask them, enquire of them. But in children it is normal, please. In adults it is not so. Now, there are people who put their hands and feet always apart, like Psorinum. They cannot sleep with their limbs close. Some like their head high. Some like the head low. Now, so much for the question of position in sleep.

I had just a patient for whom I could not see what remedy was to be given. She was a young girl of 14 years age. Can you imagine? She weighed 65 kg at 14 years of age! She was myxoedematous. When she was younger, something had happened to her in the school which she was not able to describe. Her teacher had come at her with a pen and the girl had become very much frightened. Since then she has been becoming more and more obese. She had been to every gland specialist and had taken every treatment with no result. She had also another symptom. She was always tired. She would come from school and go to bed. And it is a life which horrified her mother to see a girl coming home like that. I interrogated her much and got out one more symptom. You know we always search for the cardinal symptom. There is one symptom in everybody which is so peculiar, so extraordinary that when you find this symptom it leads you to the remedy. I call this the cardinal symptom, the pilot symptom. It is very rare that you do not find other symptoms fitting in with the remedy indicated by this cardinal symptom.

This girl was saying, "Ah, yes. I have also a kind of wheezing breathing and sometimes a little asthmatic but with this difficult breathing I am always better while lying flat." With difficult breathing people would like to sit and breath but this girl was just the contrary. We like contraries. We like things which make us reflect and say, "Stop now. This is not normal." What is the matter? She was always very chilly and I learnt that this girl always liked something warm around her, and she was not very clean I must say. And for my nose it was not the perfume of Eau de Cologne, when I went near her to look at her. All this was so plain so far as I know, that I gave her one dose of *Psor*. 10M and since that time she has already emaciated many kilograms. And now she is sleeping normally with an expression which is very much pleasant. She is so full of pep that she comes from the school to study and in the morning she says to her mother, "Please, I will go early to school because I like the school so much", and she plays with other children which she never did and when she comes home she does not go to bed to lie down, but she would like to study or to go to play outside — all with *Psor*. 10M, one dose. That is the law of homeopathy.

So, you see, we must pay attention to the symptoms. I remember another case which was very funny. It was a physician from Congo. He came to see me because he had many symptoms. The case was a little difficult, cases of physicians are always difficult. They interpret the symptoms. They tell you symptoms of this remedy and that. They always modify them. It was not very clear. But, thank God, I got one symptom, a key symptom. He told me, and it was very funny, "I can never go to the toilet without a handkerchief." "What is the matter?" "When I go to the toilet to pass my stool, I must take my handkerchief because my nose starts running." Of course, an allopath would laugh at it and may be also a homoeopath, but a good homoeopath will laugh internally, being so satisfied. This is a very good symptom, this is a pilot symptom, this is a cardinal symptom, this is a symptom that will lead to the cure because it is in the repertory. With the divine homoeopathy, you just have to open this divine book that is there (*Kent's Repertory*) and you just search and there is only one remedy for that symptom. And the only remedy is *Thuja* — the only one! You see you have to only open the repertory and you get the remedy — *Thuja*. So a funny symptom like this leading to the remedy is one of the marvels of homoeopathy. When you know a corner of the picture, you can know the whole picture. The patient is not someone you know but as you continue to ask him questions, he asks you "How do you know this, Doctor?" Of course, as I begin to open a little of the corner and look into him, I know he will have such and such symptoms though it is not someone I know. It is like a picture of a great painter, you know you can open a corner and tell what will be the rest. Of course, if it is a picture of Leonard da Vinci or Raphael, you will be knowing the rest by knowing a corner. And it is the same with homoeopathy. You know your materia medica, you open the corner and it looks like *Thuja*. Now you would like to ask, "Have you had Sycosis or gleet before?" No you must not ask such questions that he can answer by a 'Yes' or 'No'. But you must put your questions in such a way that he is free to give the answers though you may know the answer already. Yes, here in this case it was exactly *Thuja*. So as I told you, the non-pathognomonic symptom leads you to the remedy if you can discover the rather singular, the more typical, peculiar symptom as stated in paragraph 153 of the *Organon*. So this you must know absolutely.

Now, you have considered sleep — what the patient is doing during sleep with his hands, with his feet, with the head and so on. So it is a question of finding a right symptom. Now, after considering the desires and aversions, the symptoms of sleep, the general symptoms, we can go to the mental symptoms. This will be the time before going to the sexual symptoms. Because mental is alright, but sexual is something that is more difficult to ask. Mental symptoms are of a different class. Of course, as I told you, a vague symptom like sadness does not interest us a bit, but if it is sadness before menses only, or sadness only in the evening when it is twilight, or for example, there is sadness when you are thanking people or when you make a discourse, or when you cry you feel better (some others feel worse), this is interesting because it is something different. If I tell you please go to the station to meet one of my friends who is coming and he has two eyes, two ears, two legs and so on, you cannot distinguish him. But if I tell you he has a green *Topee*, he has one eye closed, he has a nose just turned to the left and he is limping, of course, you will find him quickly. It is just the way you must proceed when you are trying to find something in repertory. Try to find modalities please and symptoms which go with these. But a general symptom like sleeplessness, or sadness is no symptom.

Now, what questions shall we ask about mental symptoms? You know these symptoms are very peculiar. They really represent the patient and for us homoeopaths it is really the main thing to match or to try to match. We must know how to ask for mental symptoms. One doctor told me, the first time I was working with him, that if you are not able at the first consultation to make a patient cry or laugh, if you do not touch the heart of the patient you will not find the remedy. Now there are different questions to ask. Of course, if you ask somebody, "Tell me what are your defects please", he laughs and says he has so many. "I have so many, I cannot tell you. Ask my mother, my father, my wife". Somebody who cannot remain patient may tell you that he is absolutely patient. It is just the contrary to what they are. It is one of the funny things in life that we believe some things which are contrary to fact. We believe a patient is very kind but when we hear about him we find it is exactly the contrary. So please be very modest about what you think about yourself and try to think when you see in others some defect which makes you irritable, about your own defect, that you have exactly this defect and when you are angry about something and you feel irritated about different things that you see in somebody, they are the little things that we have exactly. But you know the subconscious likes to hide our conscious defects. So we do not know ourselves really exactly.

Now, the first question we ask a patient is this and I have found this a question which opens the situation well. "What is in your life the greatest grief that you have gone through?" So they cannot say 'Yes' or 'No'. There are some who say they have had no grief or pleasure. "You are very ungrateful. Now think," you say. Some remember the love affairs when they begin to think. Some others have lost their parents and they begin to think about that and the tears come out. Some others have lost all their fortune. People begin to think (very often they have never done it) when you ask them what is the greatest grief, and really there are many people who cry. But please do not remain long in this situation. It is not good. Very quickly you ask, "What was your greatest pleasure?" At once they dry up their tears and they think and say, "Yes. I married a very nice girl. I choose a profession which was for me my greatest pleasure", and so on.

It is more easy to save the situation and partake of the little deficiency they may have so that the patient tells you, "Yes, I have this and that." Take somebody who is jealous. Suppose, a lady is jealous of her husband who is flying in every direction with other women, you know it is normal. You will not take this as a symptom. But suppose for no reason she thinks of him the whole night. Suppose she found some odour of perfume or something like that and she tries to arrange in her imagination many things, it is interesting for us to know that she is brooding over things which are really not existing, building them up in her own imagination. So about these different reactions you can ask and find that some people are sulky while some others, when there will be trouble, just sit for one or two hours and then they accept it very well.

Then comes the very important thing, namely fears. There is in this world something which is really very intoxicating about fears. So you must know many fears. You must ask for fear of animals, fear of tunnels, fear of the future, fear of different diseases, fear of crime etc. You must be able to ask questions about these fears. You will see how it is that people have fear that you will never dream of; fears that something will happen. A lady says, "Yes, I am sure my husband will not come back today, he will have an accident". This is interesting. Of course, about fears of animals, if somebody tells you about fears of animals you must also ask, "What kind of animals?" for fear of snakes is pretty normal. So this will not count as a special fear. Regarding fear of dogs, it depends. There are people who will cross a street when they see a dog, because they fear it terribly. Some others, they have been bitten (by a dog) when they were young and they are fearing it now. Of course, this is not so important.

You must allow the patient to go through and let him have his say. If you ask them, "What are your fears?", they do not tell. Habitually they do not like to tell about their fears. Of course, that diminishes their status. So do not try. You must put it this way. "There are many people who have got fear of this and that" and she at once says "Yes" or "No". Or she will not say Yes or No. She may say, "I have fear of that." It is what you want. When you have finished your questioning, you must go back and cross-question and see again, by asking differently, if fear is the symptom, if really this symptom is there, if the symptom is correct. And sometimes unfortunately what you were so pleased to find at first, you may look and find later that it is not at all a good symptom. You see that in your sudden questioning you have made a mistake in not understanding well or you have not put the question as it should be put and so on. There are many shades that you must pay attention to. Now the fears are very important. Then comes somebody, who had told you she had no thought of suicide at all, who may now answer "I would choose a river". But if she is thinking of suicide, or she had thought of suicide before which she did not tell you, now she reveals it by answering this question.

It is just one of those cross-questions you must try to put and it is interesting. So you ask your question about suicide. But sometimes the patient is not interested in saying 'I think of suicide.' But then you can see it in the pupil, in the right pupil and not only flat representing of grief as I told you, it will be more flat. It is a suicidal tendency and (if it shows) in the right pupil, it is always something non-bloody, for example (suicide) by poison, drowning etc If in the left eye, suicide is attempted in a bloody way, for example by jumping from a height etc., always bloody, always something ugly to see. You see these marks in the pupil very long in advance. The *Aurum* will never tell you (of their intention to commit suicide) but the *Nux vomica* will tell you, at that time. "Yes, I will shoot myself or I will do this and that". But not *Aurum*.

He will hide, may be till the last moment when it is too late. But if you look in the eyes, you will know it.

Impatience, irritability — patients who go out of order because they are sensitive, they feel things too quickly and this way we must know the kind of irritability they have. They know this habitually not by themselves but from the people around them. The wife or the husband will tell you what they are. Then one symptom is very important for the discrimination, you know. It is to us very interesting, it is what we call the eliminatory symptom. We mean by this, the rubrics which will eliminate absolutely some other remedies. There are cold and hot remedies like Dr Tyler puts it. It is good. It may be very good but still you must be very sure that your are right. The patient will tell you he is chilly, the others will say he is not so chilly. Some of them may say that they do not suppose there is heat, and yet they are in a room where you are very hot enough, but they say nothing. They may come even in warm clothes. You must be careful about what they tell you. So I do not find this rubric the best one for eliminating drugs. It is a good one of course (in a negative way) e.g. when the patient, especially one whom you think is a *Sepia* patient tells you she is not chilly. Of course she cannot be *Sepia* because *Sepia* patients are very chilly. You can see that if an *Apis* patient tells you he can support the heat very well he will not need *Apis*. Just like when the patient tells you he never drinks water for *Pulsatilla* you are very pleased. But please remember if she tells you afterwards, "Yes, I am thirsty only at 2 o'clock", it is still Pulsatilla, in the first grade please. Never thirsty except at 2 o'clock! This is one of those things you must know because otherwise you may make a mistake.

There is one eliminating symptom which I find very good provided the symptom is very typical. "What is the effect of consolation?" There are patients who seek consolation and there are others who hate it. They will later tell you that it all depends from whom the consolation comes. "If it is my sweetheart consoling me or my wife or my mother, I like it very much, not the people whom I do not like very much." So with this answer it is amelioration by consolation because really they are ameliorated. You must not take this amelioration by consolation as a symptom. But there are people who really say, "When I am upset, I go into my room". *Ignatia*, *Arsenic*, *Nux vomica* and such remedies cover this aversion to consolation. And in this way it is very good to use as an eliminating symptom. There are few such eliminating symptoms. If somebody hates consolation, it is a good symptom. If somebody likes sweets and he is a young boy, it is not a symptom. Everybody likes candies. So when there are plenty of people with the same symptom, do not consider this as very important.

And amelioration by consolation is not a symptom to be taken in the repertory. And why he (Kent) has put it there was because everybody was saying so and he could not avoid it. There may be a state where you find that amelioration by consolation is something very curious e.g. a patient has sciatica, a patient has terrible headache and consolation ameliorates. This is very interesting. There *Pulsatilla* may come in because it is something you will not expect and because it is something not usual. You must interpret the materia medica as it is. What is rare, what is peculiar, what is strange, this is the thing you must remember.

I remember a professor, well-known in Geneva, who suffered from asthma. Nobody could cure him. He went to homoeopath, allopath, naturopath, etc. Ultimately he came to see me. It was very difficult to find the remedy. The symptoms were simply pathognomonic. I saw some signs in his eyes and in his writing and I was so struck that I told him, "Sometimes there are symptoms very difficult to express but you know in homoeopathy we always consider the disposition of the patients something sacred, which I am not there to judge. I am there merely to comprehend, to help the human heart as Kent says and in this spirit we can help sometimes very much". So I tried to look aside, not to look at him. He said, "Yes, I will tell you something," and so out he came with many things. "You know, I have a terrible habit. Every Sunday I take the train to Luzerne. Why every Sunday? Because there are many people in the train with their children. And I choose a compartment where there are many ladies with their children. And I choose a place where there are little girls and I come near the lady and take the girl over my knees and I rock her to and fro, and this excites me splendidly. I am very much pleased.. So, every Sunday I go to Luzerne ten times you know, going and coming, and try to find people to excite me. Can you imagine this? And when I go to a hotel, I always choose a room not inside but outside, where there are other houses opposite and I like to undress myself when their window is open, so that the people can see me? This also excites me. Can you imagine this? Or I ring the bell for my breakfast and the moment the lady brings the breakfast I just take my shirt out so that I am almost naked." You know how funny it is. He is an exhibitionist and it is very hard to know this. And in the repertory there is a rubric for this. Where is this rubric? It is not given under the word exhibitionist. That is the trouble. When somebody is like that, what is he? He is shameless, so it is under the rubric "Shameless, exposes the person." Exactly, there is *Phosphorus* there. *Phosphorus* was the remedy. This, I gave him and his asthma went beautifully away. In this case I did not think of his asthma. I think of the symptom more important than asthma. Asthma was a result of this thing, it was the outward expression. But this symptom he never told anybody, because he was a professor, you know. And when he told me I put it right with *Phos*. And the result was splendid.

When your patient is homosexual, where do you search in the repertory? It is a very interesting symptom (Someone in the audience "Increased sexuality"). No, no. It is not increased sexuality, not at all. This is a mental symptom. You must learn your repertory by heart almost and know where to search. You know, I am looking into the repertory for the last forty seven years, every day you know, fifty times at least. Of course, you will never forget it when you find it once, if you have the grey substance beside the white one (in the brain). Look what is written 'Love, love with one of her own sex'. It is interesting. Of course, I have added and corrected my repertory, because

I am now reading much *Knerr's Repertory* which is a very fine book. So I find *Pulsatilla* in my repertory. So about the sexual symptoms, your situation is like that because it depends whether it is a lady or a gent. It is more easy to ask questions of a lady than a man. It is very funny but for a lady doctor it is more easy to ask questions of a man than of a lady. It is a question of confidence. We don't like to tell our weaknesses to someone of the same sex.

Now in the mental symptoms also you must be very cautious. You may ask questions about the sexual functions. It is normal, everybody tells. You say, "but there are people who would like to have intercourse every day or twice a day." "No", he says, "it is not so much". "How much?" "Once a month or once in two months". I am astonished to know this. "Why so?" "Because", he says, "I don't feel like it, because I am tired," and now he tells you, "I have no good erections". Now you begin to know he is impotent. That is why he does not like to have it often. Or if it is a woman they tell you, "Oh, I have aversion to it. I like my husband. He is lovely but the moment I come towards him, I almost feel to cry because I feel I cannot have an intercourse. I must enjoy it, but I cannot. I must play the act all the time." So, you see, you begin to know that what it is. You may say also "There are some people who when they were young were excited." "Yes" the patient says "I was also like that." You always give the example of somebody else. So they will tell you all about themselves. I had a patient. He had convulsions in the midst of coition. This is a rare symptom. We have a remedy for this (*Bufo*).

I had another one who wets his bed regularly with prostatic fluid or semen and whenever he goes to his wife, he has erection alright but not one drop of semen comes. It is curious, is it not? There are others who have blood coming instead of semen. So you may ask such questions and you begin to know some of the things.

A lady with *Sepia* or *Causticum* symptoms but who is very much excited for intercourse is not a *Sepia* or *Causticum*. You have made a mistake in interrogation for it is *Sepia*, *Bromium* or *Causticum* where you know they hate intercourse. And in this way it is interesting.

It is true that besides the homoeopathic remedy, Chinese acupuncture helps very much in those cases. Of course, when you do homoeopathy, do your homoeopathy. I hate mixing any other pathy, because it interferes with homoeopathy in a way. You must avoid any other therapeutics and remedies, but when you use any other way of tackling the patient, either by massage or by osteopathy or things of that kind or by acupuncture, you are using therapeutics which help it. Acupuncture is the Chinese method of touching the seven hundred and twelve points that are in the body, where the resistance of the skin is less and where currents of energy, vital energy, are flowing out at different points. You must know these points. It is a very hard question, a question of memory which is terrible because you must know the names of the points in Chinese and their number, where it is situated and so on. But it is interesting. The patient comes, for example with some disorder that is also difficult to cure with homoeopathy. She comes with a severe pain and is unable to lift the arm. She cannot, you know, comb her hair in the morning. But you just prick on another part of the body, perhaps in the foot at a certain point. You see suddenly she can move, not tomorrow or an hour later but at once! The moment you prick she can do this. Sometimes it holds for ever, sometimes you must come in (and repeat it) after eight days again but the result is so quick, so amazing, so astonishing, like your remedy. If the pain is on the right hand side, if it is on the cubital side, if the pain is in the front or middle, according to this we may prick different places on the foot, but when it is on the other side, we must use a golden needle. And it depends, you know, also on the direction of the prick, whether you turn it to the right or left side, whether you prick two times or one time slowly, if you prick first a little and then you go down quickly and soon. This is not a question of psychological effect in hysterical patients. Unfortunately, if you don't touch them at the right point the effect is nil, but if you prick at the right point the effect is like that of the homoeopathic remedy. You can give your hysterical patients many remedies, but there is nothing, no effect. But the moment you give them the right remedy they are cured. So is the case with acupuncture. An asthmatic comes to you gasping for breath. You prick him on the right point and he will suddenly say, "Oh, I can breathe." It is marvellous. But when you have not touched the right point there is no result.

Then this question of hysteria. I am sorry to say in my 45 years of practice I have never found a hysterical patient inventing a disease. As Hahnemann said the patient may exaggerate the symptoms or diminish his feelings. But patients who invent all their symptoms, I have never seen. Exaggeration, diminution, sometimes falsification. Yes. But inventing the whole disease I have never seen. So you see about hysteria. I have never used this rubric (hysteria) in the repertory. It is very easy to speak of hysteria like we speak of rheumatism, when we do not know anything about the disease. So we use the words wrongly.

HOMOEOPATHIC CASE TAKING: SOME POINTS

There are three cavities in the body containing organs, the *first* one being the head, the most noble one because it protects the capital of the man. It is, of course, his capital, his millions of dollars which are there, it is his friend, his intelligence and his work. It is very thick. It has only small apertures, as in a bank, you know, one or two windows. The *second* one is the chest. It is made of flesh and bone. You can look through it, you can see through as in a jail. This contains the heart, the lungs, and the different organs, the thymus and so on. The *third* one is the abdomen. It has no wall and has nothing before that. It has only muscles, but no bones to protect. Here, only on one side it is protected. With an umbrella you can pierce it if you like. So thus is the third one.

And what is interesting? The first one contains the brain which is working at our will. We can do what we like. This is ours to command. But here in the chest, we cannot command very much. We can breath more quickly, we can breath more slowly, but we cannot stop breathing for 20 hours. And the heart, you can try to make it work more quickly, but you cannot command your heart like you will. So there the commands are not so important. But here in the abdomen you can command nothing. Here every organ works by itself while you sleep, like the regulation of the temperature which keeps you at 37°C, the organs responsible for digestion, for urination etc., everything goes on working without our will.

Now the Lord arranges everything in such a way that every part of the body reveals also the total, every small part reveals the whole. The face, for example, can be divided into three different parts: the eyes and the part above it, the part between the eyes and the lips and the part below that. Here, in the first part, you have the eye and the forehead. When you are angry, you frown (the forehead furrows). So also, with your eyes. You can face somebody and fire somebody, or you can make sweet eyes (winking), you know. Now these are all connected with the brain.

Then in the second part, there is the nose. In serious disease, the nose is flapping, for example in the lung disease. Or, with the heart disease, you can see a little telengiectasis or blue vessels visible on the side of the nose.

And the third one is the mouth. And the mouth and the lips can say many things. Big bulging lips express people who are very greedy for eating, good eating; also for love, because you kiss with the lips. This corresponds to the genital parts. Only by looking at the face, you may know everything in the body. There are people who by looking at the hand or at the nails can tell you everything and some of them by the form of teeth. They can tell you everything from the skull. One of my pupils had discovered that the ear is the inverse of the foetus and that there you have the vertebral column above, and below that the eyes and the nose, then you have skin. There you have the geographical map of the whole body in the ear, and by touching certain points with the needle, sometimes you can cure things at once. Ladies who have always tiresome backaches, who always have a pain there, just touch them near the corner of the ear there, very near point 4 of 5 and 2, and when you touch it, the pain which they have had for 4 or 5 weeks sometimes disappears. Now they have no pains. In 10 seconds the pain has gone. Repeat after 8 days, sometimes not. It is amazing, but I have not the time today to speak to you about the marvellous method of acupuncture.

Now, I told you listen, observe, write. After this comes examination. Examine the patient carefully. Examine your patient with all the modern ways, with most modern methods. For what purpose? Of course, you may say for diagnosis, if you like to please yourself. But in reality, this is very important for you, for your homoeopathic diagnosis.

As Kent says, when you write down the symptoms, divide your page into two parts. In one, you write your pathognomonic symptoms and in the other there, your non-pathognomonic symptoms. When a man comes with a cough and says there is a pain there when he coughs, with sputum which is yellow, anything about the cough, you write it here. But when he tells you, for example, there is a chill in his left leg when he is coughing or that he has a headache when he is coughing or that he has any curious symptom that you do not know why he has it, we put it there on the other side, on the non-pathognomonic side.

Now I remember the story of Dr Charette. He wrote a very interesting book, "*What is Homoeopathy*?". If you have not read it, you should read this because it is very amusing and full of funny things. But what is interesting? One day a doctor came to him and told him, "You know, I have been treated for three months. I have a terrible vertigo, a very curious giddiness every time I read the paper. The more I read, the more I have my giddiness and you know I cannot read any book, I cannot read any paper. I am very cross. I went to the specialists who put me on the whirling chair and tried to find out what is wrong with me. They could not diagnose what is the disease. They looked into my ears. They looked into my throat. They found nothing.

They gave me massage, they gave me electricity, but you know I still have the vertigo. What to do?" And now it is so simple for a homoeopath. If a remedy has ever produced giddiness while reading, you can cure this patient. Now, sometimes, I feel you can make the diagnosis of the disease also by knowing the remedy, and you can know the other symptoms. So Dr S; tried to do something which is sometimes tedious but he said, "I am sure this is in the materia medica". He did not know anything about it, but he tried to put this affirmation. "But when and where, I do not know, I will search and I will read all of Hahnemann's materia medica from beginning to end until I find the remedy for this vertigo." The physician thought it was a very nice way of course. If it had been in the letter "S" it would have taken many months. But you know the Lord is so marvellous and kind, it was in the letter "A", but not at the beginning of the letter "A". Otherwise it could have been *Aconite*, *Agnus castus*, or *Ailanthus glandulose*, *Allium cepa* or *Ammonium carbonicum* or something like that. It was at the end of the letter "A" and by turning the pages it took something like seven hours for Dr S. The remedy was Arnica but when you find Arnica for a case with a curious symptom like that, you think there must be trauma. He asked his patient, "Have you ever had any trouble, something like an accident?" "No, no, never". But when he persisted, "Do you ever remember having had an accident?" He said "Yes. One day I was asked early in the morning to see an emergency case. I did not have my car. I took a taxi and I told him to go quickly, *Jaldhi*, *Jaldhi*[4] to the place and you know I went to the car and we came into a road where there was a little depression, and so I bumped my head against the top of the vehicle. And since that time I have vertigo." So homoeopathy knows when you have vertigo, and it corresponds to Arnica, you must have had trauma. It is curious that you can thus make the diagnosis and have the remedy. But you know, it would

---

4. *Hindi word for quickly*

have been easier if the doctor would have known the use of the repertory. If you take Vertigo and search under the rubric you will find 'Vertigo aggravated by reading'. There are many remedies here. But what is interesting? There is only one remedy which has Vertigo on reading a long time and that remedy is Arnica. There are other remedies for other kinds of reading e.g. for reading aloud there is still another remedy. You know, you are learning a lot of things by studying the repertory. So everybody must possess a repertory besides the *Organon*, besides his materia media and besides he will have his memory in the first cavity (head), you know so that you will be able to find the remedy very quickly.

So much about the value of symptoms. Now examine your patient thoroughly. You, of course, know what are the symptoms which are pathognomonic. Do not take them into consideration first. Take them last. If the patient has pain in the knee, pain in the eye, pain or trouble in the right arm, don't care about it. You don't throw it away, no. But set it aside simply. And if he has any symptoms which are funny, like the symptoms of the nose, like the symptoms of giddiness, funny symptoms,, of course, these you must take into consideration first. You put it down and you begin to study first your non-pathognomonic symptoms; and your best cures will always be done with the non-pathognomonic symptoms. Now, if you have very few symptoms you must take what is available, then you must take the pathognonomonic symptoms. But the more you can take care of those others (non-pathognomonic) the better will be the cure. Forget the disease, see the patient, see the symptoms which he predicated of himself. These will help you to find the right remedy better than anything else.

Now comes the time you must co-ordinate. The fifth stage is co-ordination. This is the stage to co-ordinate the symptoms, to establish the value of symptoms, to weigh. It is a question of quantity for the allopath while for the homoeopath it is a question of quality because homoeopathy is a method of quality.

Now when you have symptoms, what are the types of symptoms that are most important? It is not the question of taking down all the symptoms of the patient, page after page. As Dr Weir has very well said, "Take the minimum symptoms of maximum importance". What are the symptoms that are most important? There are exactly five categories of symptoms. If you remember this, and if you take care of this, you will make beautiful cures.

First the mind symptoms, providing they are important, they are characteristic. If the patient says, "I have not good memory, I am sad very often. I am a little dull, I cannot concentrate myself". There are 500 remedies for each one of these symptoms and it is not very interesting. If you go to the station to search for a friend or somebody you do not know who is arriving, and he wrote to you I have two eyes, one nose, two legs and one head, you will not recognise him, but if it is a lady with the green hat, she is squinting, you know, she is limping and she has a white handkerchief in her hand, then you will recognise her at once. So the question is to know the characteristic symptoms and to know what the symptoms that predicate the patient. So you have typical symptoms, I do not have the time today to tell you all the gradations into the mind's symptoms. It is fascinating to know about the many symptoms of the intellect, which are the ones that are more important, and which are the ones that are less important. But you will always have symptoms of fear or symptoms of excitation, irritability or weeping, sadness or despair and so on. Always it is possible to find such symptoms.

Now the *second*, I can indicate this way, the omega[5] this is the general symptom. The general symptoms in the repertory are in the last chapter because the repertory is thus made, first the intellect, last the general symptoms and in between sandwiched all the rest. You have all the symptoms coming from the head down, between the intellect and the general. And remember that the general symptoms are those of aggravation by heat or cold, aggravation by different seasons, aggravation by the weather, by the position, by going to the mountains, or near the seashore, by resting, by dozing and you know there are plenty of others. Most materiopathic influences are general symptoms which affect the whole body and not only one part. So you have the general symptoms.

Then comes here, the symptoms of the stomach, not of the digestion and so on, but about the aversions and cravings. This is a very important thing. When you ask someone, "Do you like sweet, or do you like bitter things?",

5. *The last letter of the Greek alphabet meaning here the last chapter in "Kent's Repertory".*

if he says “Yes, I like them” or “I do not like them” (in a monotonous tone), this is not important. But when you ask, “What about salt?”, you see his eyes become bright. He likes it so much that even before tasting the soup, he puts salt in it. Se he has a craving for salt. People who cannot do without going to sweetmeat merchants for buying sweet things and delicacies, pastries, etc., it is a desire, a craving for sweets. Now there are people who eat salads you know with vinegar. When it is finished, they put a little vinegar in a spoon and take it, so much they like sour things. In the morning they take a lemon and they take it raw as such, so much they like it. So you see this is a craving.

Now, an aversion. If somebody makes a face, really it is a disgust, (he means) “No, I do not like it”. You must note the expression on the face as well as the words expressed by the patient. So you have there the symptoms of cravings or desires.

Now this is a rubric that is very important — amelioration and aggravation by certain items of food. There are people who like very much food with cream and sugar and sweet, but they are sick right after, no matter how much they like it. So they may have a craving for it and an aggravation from it. If you have an aggravation from something you like, it is curious. But to this, you must be at once attentive. When you have a patient in acute and very serious stage and his life is in danger, if he craves something, give it to him. But in chronic cases keep it away. So if somebody likes alcohol in a chronic case, he says when I drink brandy I feel so well, you must prohibit it. If in an acute disease he is dying and he wants brandy, give it to him.

Now you have after this the sleep symptoms. The sleep symptoms are very important because when you are asleep you do not know what you are doing and sleep for a physician and a homoeopathic physician is very important. First, the position in sleep. It seems to be very funny but there are people who sleep on the abdomen, on their stomach. Why, I do not know, but it is a very good symptom of *Medorrhinum*, *Pulsatilla* and other remedies. And I know there are people who cannot sleep on the left side. Some others who have heart disease can only lie on the left side. Some of those sleep like that with hands above the head, you know. The children must sleep like that. But when an adult sleeps like that, he may be having liver disease. There are people with asthma who are always better when lying flat. Why? Explain it to me. It is very good non-pathognomonic symptom because we cannot explain it. So remember the position in sleep.

Now what are you doing when you are sleeping? There are people who keep their eyes open. It is funny but it is so. Or they keep their eyes half-closed with the eye-balls going up. So you take notice of this of course. Now there are people who squint when they sleep. But some others make a motion like this (chewing). This is *Bryonia*. Of course, when a child is making a motion like a rabbit, it is always *Bryonia* in delirium sometimes or in fever. Now there are people who chatter in sleep. Some of them grind their teeth, some of them clench their teeth as if they do not like to open, as in trismus or tetanus. There are people who talk. There are people who shriek. There are people who sing. Some of them weep. It is interesting to watch somebody in sleep when you can find so many symptoms. There are people who slide down the bed by morning. Well, you see these things are interesting. When they slide down like this habitually, they sleep with their jaws open and this is a very good symptom of *Muriatic acid*. Every body knows it. So you can see by looking at the different states of the sleep you can learn a lot. Now the sleep can be restless, it can be comatose, it can be semiconscious. You know the different kinds of sleep. There are restless people who always roll up and down. In the morning they must search for the different pieces of the bedding around them. Others remain exactly as they were. You can find all these in the repertory. Open the repertory and you will learn a lot. By turning the pages you find different things, they correspond to certain remedies out of which you can choose.

Then there is sleepiness. Some people are sleepy in the daytime; when they are listening to a lecture, they just begin to doze. There are people who cannot listen or go to a lecture without closing their eyes, or they begin to sleep after lunch. There was a notary. When he was writing what the client had said to him, he was in what we call a narcolepsy. It was a terrible heaviness of his eyes, sleepiness. He could not help closing his eyes. It was a disease. Of course, *Opium* will help him.

Then there are people who are sleepless. Sleeplessness can be in the beginning of the night. It can be in the second part of the night. It can be from 1 to

2, from 2 to 3, from 4 to 5 and these are indications for different remedies. When in the morning it is *Natrum sulph*. When it is from 2 to 3 or 1 to 2, it can be *Kali carb.*, *Kali ars.*, and so on. Everybody knows those little shades. There are people who are very sleepy. They cannot keep their eyes open in the evening, but the moment they are in the bed they cannot sleep. This is very often *Ambra* or such other remedies. Open your repertory and read. You must have the *Organon*, materia medica and a repertory plus your brain which helps you.

Now come the dreams. There are dreams which are repeating every time. There are dreams which are prophetic. The moment they dream something, the next day it will happen. The patient begins to dream one day and then it continues all the week like in a cinema. It is funny but there are people you know, who have dreams that are exhausting e.g. as if they are climbing mountains. In the morning they are all covered with sweat and they feel so tired. All this is found in the repertory. Open your repertory. See such of these things.

And to finish the last about this. This is co-ordination. Co-ordination of the sexual symptoms. Of course, this requires the tact and the delicacy of thought of the physician to talk of this question with the patient.

You will never begin with this. If you know how to handle human hearts and human beings, they will tell you very easily their troubles, especially their sexual troubles, that they will hide from everybody else. You must know if the patient is plus or minus, whether he has hyper or exaggerated feeling of sex or the other one, no feeling or aversion. You will know also deviations and abnormal possibilities. You will know many more things. I have not the time to tell you today. By looking at the patient you can know many things that he will not tell you, I see very much my corneal microscope. I can know at once if the patient has onanism, masturbation, if he is much excited, if a lady is a virgin or not and so on. I can know from the eyes many of the impulses of the human being but I have not the time today to expose this to you all. It is very complicated. But one thing I will tell you. In this part comes for the lady everything pertaining to the menses. But what interests us, it is not only to know about the menses, if the colour is dark or the colour is pale or reddish, but also if it is in clots, irritating the parts or if it is offensive or if it is bland or about the quality of the blood, if it is more at night or more in day time, more in the morning — if it stains the linen, if they are yellow or of different colours and so on. You may find in the repertory all the answers for these questions. This is very important. Now you have, you know, with the repertory and with your Organon, many things to ponder over, and I think with all these explanations you will be able to feel the enthusiasm, that I feel for homoeopathy.

Because the more an allopath grows old the less he believes in his medicines. In a trolley car, when you see two physicians, one an allopath and one a homoeopath, you know what they think. One thinks of the leg of the patient which will be in the anatomy, pathological anatomy, whether is can be cut off to cure disease. If it is of the abdomen whether there is a tumour and so on. Well, he thinks of negative. But the homeopath is always smiling and thinking what remedy may I find for this patient, there may be a remedy for this patient, may be we will be able to save this patient. Mostly he always thinks with hope, there is always the possibility of learning something more. The more an allopath grows old, the more he is pessimistic; the more the homoeopath grows old, the more he is enthusiastic and optimistic.

SOME SERIOUS CASES

I will give you a short survey of some serious cases. Of course, there is no need to tell you that it is possible to help such patients, with homoeopathy. I will not tell the 14 cases I have prepared. It is too long.

It was in the best University in America, may be the best in the world, the California University, where they had decided to have a Chair for Homoeopathy and the Professor elected to the Chair was a German who was very intelligent. He came before his confreres. He told them, "I do not wish that you should send me the case you think you will be able to help. I would like you to send me those cases that you can do nothing about, the cases that you cannot help or that you have treated for months or may be years and are still there chronic, and there are chronic infirmities. So if you could send those I will see what I can do". And he received three cases.

The *first* was from a Professor of Dermatology who told him, "That is very nice. I can send you a case of

Verruca obstinata. It is a case of warts that I have treated now for one year, and this man has 26 horny, very large warts. He is 20 years of age, and for one year I have tried caustics, acid, X-ray, etc. I have even tried surgery but when I take one out, another comes in its place to laugh at me". So, he was very cross. "I do not want to see this man when he comes. Now, I have told my assistant that I have had enough of him". Thereupon, the homoeopath studied the case. It was a case of *Thuja*. He gave the patient *Thuja* 200 and you know, the disease, which had lasted for one to one and a half years, disappeared in two weeks, beautifully and quickly, and it never came again. (Applause).

The *second* one was a funny case. It was the case of a surgeon. This surgeon was very skilful and he was getting a little old at 65 years, and whenever he was stitching, every time he was stitching up the intestine, suddenly his middle finger would bend down like that, down like a spring, and he had to push it up. When he continued the stitching, promptly it would go down like that again. It is very amusing but in the pathology what are you doing with this? Go to your Pharmacist and ask him what he will give for a spring finger? So one day, there was a handful of blood coming out on the operation table and he was saying, "Now, I must abandon my profession because, this makes me so furious, but I do not know what to do." And his assistants were just crying with him and they were telling him, "We do not know what to tell you". At that moment, my brother who was my first pupil, who is now in California, San Francisco, was passing there and one of them jokingly said, "Ha! Here is a homoeopath. Let us ask him what he can do". It was a joke, you know but it was a challenge too. My brother came in and said "What is the matter? Oh, I see! Very simple". Although there were no symptoms, you know, only this, my brother studied the case and he gave one dose of *Ruta* 200 and since that time the finger was very obedient and never came down again. (Cheers).

Now, the *third* case, the whole hospital came to know of this case of the professor and they were very cross, and there was one, the Professor of Opthalmology, who said, "I have a case for you. This, you will not be able to cure". It is a disease of the gland. I do not know whether you know of this disease, a disease with a very complicated name. It was a man of Spain who discovered this disease of the gland. It is a disease affecting the gland, of the eye that secrete the tears for ladies, you know and of men too, which are coming regularly into the eye, to wash the dirt, to clean the eye, and to keep the cornea always in good vitality. Now, this gland dries up. No more tears and the patient's eyes begin to become very painful. Inflammation begins, gangrene sometimes supervenes. It is sometimes very serious, threatening his life. They do not know what to do. They try vitamins. They try many things, all in vain.

Now, this patient was very funny, she had very funny symptoms. She had trouble first on the left side. Second, generally she desired all the time to take oysters. She was very fond and had a craving for oysters. She liked pickles very much. Now she could not support the odour of tobacco. That is, when somebody was smoking she cannot remain in the same room, it was unbearable. Now when she had perspiration, the linen was becoming always yellow. Funny, yellow when she perspired. Besides these, it was impossible for her to find the nourishment which was cold enough or hot enough. She could not support anything either too cold or too hot. She was always eating something tepid. But too hot or too cold was embarrassing and it was absolutely impossible for her to eat salad with vinegar. So all those symptoms everybody knows, are typical of *Lachesis*, *Lachesis trigonocephalus* or *Lachesis mutus*, you all know. Now for this patient, my brother gave her one dose of the 10,000th dynamisation. And what was funny, you know, she had a little aggravation after being better for three days. She began to be aggravated. On the 12th day, he repeated, which we do not do frequently, because we wait longer, but he gave her a second dose. After the second week, the patient became better and better and after a few weeks, she was completely cured. The tears came back again, redness, dryness everything disappeared. She went to the clinic and she was shown to the professor. He was spell-bound and did not know what to say.

Thus, you know, the trouble began. Since that day, can you imagine, no professor, no specialist ever again sent a case to the homoeopath. This was too dangerous! Of course, it was too dangerous to let them prove that homoeopathy is superior to any other pathy. And in this way, this school, which had to conduct a course of materia medica, had no patient to present to the class.

Now, I will not tell you all the other cases. But I will also tell you the case of my mother, because it was of someone who was very dear to me, and, I think, that it will interest you. I will tell you two cases only.

I will not speak to you of all the cases which are so frequent that at midnight, exactly at midnight, the telephone rings. In a month I may say two or three times the telephone rings at midnight. You take the telephone and a mother tells you, "Oh, Doctor! Can you come?" You hear the terrible shrieking on the telephone. Baby was shrieking because the baby had pain in the ear. What is it? It is midnight. The child is restless. His face is red and the mother does not know what to do. The child is shrieking with pain. Now what to do? Every patient who comes to me goes back with a bottle of *Aconite napellus* 200 in his pocket. I tell the mother, "Have you got *Aconite*?" Oh yes, because I give this for the cold. For the beginning of the cold, for everything which comes on suddenly, everything that comes on especially at midnight, any inflammation in appendix, or the ear, eye, anything where it is sudden, like a storm in good weather, coming suddenly. Everything which is sudden, comes suddenly and when there is restlessness, when there is anxiety, when there is thirst, when there is especially redness of the parts, think of *Aconite*. So I tell them, "You have got *Aconite*? Yes. Put a few globules in a glass of water. Give a teaspoon every five minutes. And if after 15 minutes the child still shrieks, will you phone me again?" And since 4 years I was never called a second time after midnight. The proof of the pudding is in the eating and there, I tell you, the pudding is very nice because it comes in nice little globules. And now you see, I come in the morning. Either I see a little blood, if it was haemorrhagic or a little pus, or there is nothing for the inflammation has subsided. The child is quiet. The indication is given of another remedy according to the quality of the pus — if it is red over the ear, if it is of bad odour, colour, consistency etc. Everything is in the repertory. You have only to open the page and look at it and you see, you find your remedy and you can cure the patient very easily.

Now I had a very funny case one morning. I would like to know what the allopaths would have done that morning. I know because they have tried. It was a case, a very curious case, of a man. You know, he was a janitor of the conservatory of music — a very stout man who liked to eat well, always sitting in his chair, taking telephone calls for different plays, piano or anything like that. This man is loved by everybody because he was a very jolly and nice and this man — he was 40 years or something — he had a friend, a very dear friend. He was beginning his work only at 9 o'clock. Every morning at 8 o'clock sharp he was going to the lake which is just ten minutes' walk, and taking his boat and rowing for half an hour or so with his friend. One was paddling and the other telling some story. And the friend was always very punctual. And one morning at 8 o'clock the friend was not there. So he took the phone at 5 minutes after 8, and when he heard his friend's wife on the telephone he said, "This is terrible, you know. Charles is very lazy, he is a bad boy. I hate him. He was always very regular" and so on and you know, he began quarrelling over the phone. Of course, the lady could not answer a word. He was talking himself all the time, but after a while he stopped and said, "What is the matter?" She said, "You know, my dear friend, you will not see him again". "What? I will not see him! He must come up at once". "Because he died in the night" she said. Now then, he put the telephone down and he began to hear in his right ear a terrible buzzing, so hard that he could not answer the telephone, so strong it was. He went, of course, to the doctor, who tried everything, massage, hot and cold injections, everything, but unfortunately it was impossible to cure. He was growing worse and began to be sad, melancholy. He said, "What is life going to be? I have lost my friend, and now I am almost crazy with noise". It was a case, just a hard case for homoeopathy, like other cases which are lost by the others. What is interesting is to know about the symptoms, mental symptoms, general symptoms and so on. There is one symptom above all, I forgot to tell you, above the main symptom, above all other symptoms. This is what we call the etiological symptom. If you know, after a grief or after a sudden indignation, or after anger or after an emotion somebody has been sick, you are dealing with the mind. You are not dealing with mice or guinea pigs, you are dealing with human beings, they can tell you what they feel. So I gave him the remedy for ailments from indignation and grief. At this time, it was silent grief, because he could not weep, and the only remedy which fitted him, because he was never thirsty, was *Gelsemium sempervirens.* I gave the 10M, one dose — and you know, since then, two days after the dose, he had none of the buzzing and it was for all his life finished. He had not a single noise in his ear. And the case was so fascinating and everybody was so astonished to see that this man had, for more than a year, buzzing in the ear and within a few days, it had disappeared with *Gelsemium.* It is the remedy for any trouble that comes on after grief, silent grief, combined with indignation, because he was indignant that his friend did not come it time.

Now before I finish, I will tell you the case of my mother. I will tell you the case of my mother because it is very interesting. You know, my mother was 89 years old last year. And this is the time when we must think about her departure. When one day I came home I found her in her bed, snoring, comatose; she remained thus for 8 days, without a stool, without sweat, or a drop of urine, a body, a corpse in bed, just living, pulse rather slow, pupils small, absolutely like a corpse or cadaver. I thought, of course, this was the end of her life. I would have been very pleased if she can pass away in this way, without knowing any pain. I was very pleased this way. But I was very sorry in the other way. One of my nieces who was young, who was studying Medicine said, "Why should we not give here some cortisone or injections or blood-letting, something modern?" I said, "No. I will not give my mother anything which will aggravate her situation. Now she is in such a stage. I think she is at the end but if there is any hope it must be only homoeopathy". When you have before you a body which is doing nothing, no sweating, nothing, you think of only one remedy — *Opium*. *Opium* just covers the situation. So I gave her in the corner (of the mouth) there, a few globules of *Opium* 10,000. Ten minutes later, I saw a blinking of the left eye. Half an hour later, the other eye also started blinking. She looked at me, she could not speak. The next day, she could move an arm, after a few days she was able to move her feet; she could not talk but by and by, everything was better and better everyday and in two months she was picking flowers in the mountains and helping in the kitchen. (Cheers).

Now my last case. I must take a case where really one should see whether homoeopathy is really the remedy for children, and not merely for those who believe in it and for those just psychic cases. You know, I was knowing a young assistant of a Professor of Surgery in a hospital, a very good Professor in a marvellous clinic in Paris. He had an assistant of his who was interested in homoeopathy. One day his wife had a child and a few days later she hardness of the breast, fever and pain at 12 o'clock. She asked me what to do. He was preparing to open (incise) it and I came and I found there was hardness and it was better from pressing, and I gave *Bryonia* 10M. The next morning, no pain, no fever, and in two days, she was able to give her breast to her child, and everything was over. So much touched and pleased was he that he said, "I will be pleased if you will help my children also." I said, "Sure" and gave him different remedies and he tried homoeopathy with much success.

Now, one day a boy of 10 years came at the outdoor of the polyclinic. He came with his parents, because his parents found that he had often pain in the abdomen. His mother was fearing appendix and so I examined him and I found there was really nothing, only a little tenderness. There was no case for opening the abdomen and I said he can come again after a few days or a few month when there was something more important. A few days afterwards, at midnight, the child came with his parents, unconscious, belly absolutely rigid with peritonitis. We had to open it at once and when we had opened the abdomen, a jet of pus was coming out of the opening — the abdominal cavity full of pus. It was perforated appendix. This, we see sometimes. So, with our new wonderful medicines, you know, *Penicillin*, *Streptomycin*, in and out of the body, by mouth, injection etc., within 3 days the child was well and the parents came and thanked the professor. They said they were very pleased. He said, "I think the child is saved and I am very pleased at the modern way of therapeutics and the weapons we have now to fight microbes." This was all right. Now one day later, the child was not so well. He could not eat anything or tolerate any liquid because he was vomiting at once. So he began to emaciate. After some days there was complete disintegration, and he could not eat, he could not drink. They tried to give an enema. But he could not support it. It was coming out. They tried to give an injection of glucose, different preparations you know, solutions and so on. It was causing a swelling there and was remaining like that. No absorption. Then they became desperate. So I was called in. The boy could not speak. The poor one had emaciated much, he had high fever and the case seemed lost. There was septicaemia. So the professor called the parents and said, "I am very sorry. I did my best, but the infection came again. We have tried everything. I can do nothing more; the child is probably lost. We tried even at 10 o'clock and then again at 4 o'clock. We tried to give an injection of *Penicillin* but the child is only 10 years of age and his veins are very small. We must make an incision there and find it and so on; it is very difficult."

One of his assistants was my pupil. So at 4 o'clock after the professor's visit, he phoned to me and said, "Doctor, I am so sorry about this child, I have taken him to my heart. I have tried my best. I was so pleased to see him get well and now he is going from bad to worse and he is lost. Have you any advice? Anything whatever that I can do to help him"? Surely, homoeopathy has so many weapons. But it was not a case to be laughed at. It was a very serious case. I said the first thing, you give him *Arnica montana* 10,000. Why *Arnica*? Because there is zymotic disease, there is infection, there is trauma (by surgery), because he has been opened up — Trauma. The remedy for trauma is habitually *Arnica*. So, *Arnica* may help him. It is a marvellous remedy. Give him *Arnica* at 4 o'clock today and tomorrow in the morning when he wakes up, give him one dose of *Pyrogenium* 10M. Like William Tell in Switzerland who was asked by the terrible man in Austria (Gessler) to put an apple over the head of his son, and to shoot it with one arrow, you know, the Swiss homoeopaths are also like that (sharp shooters) when they give one dose of the remedy. So in the evening at 10 o'clock the professor asked his assistants to try to give him an injection of *Penicillin*. Others were not keen because they knew what it was to go into the vein of a boy of 10 years. Besides this, they had done that before. He was not absorbing *Penicillin*. So they said, "What is the use, beginning this again? Only to satisfy the parents? To say, we have done something? But this is very wrong." So he said he will come and see the patient at 10 o'clock for the first time in many days, the patient was asleep. They said, "Sleep is a very good boon. So let him sleep till tomorrow morning." And the assistant said to the nurse, "Give him the powder tomorrow at 6 o'clock". At 6 o'clock the nurse gave him the powder, *Pyrogenium* at 9 o'clock or 10 o'clock when the professor came with his assistants and you know, the corps of the ballet with him, he went into the room with all the white shirts to look at the patient, he found the child smiling and saying, "Please give me something to drink." But the nurse said, "I will not give him something to drink because I know at once he will again vomit." The Professor said, "Try it". So they gave him a tiny half-spoon of water. They put it into the mouth and he was so pleased and everyone was so pleased they were looking with their mouth open, and it was not vomited. He asked for more and then he drank the whole glass, you know. After this they tried to give him a little milk. He could retain this very well and can you believe, two days later the drain was removed, for there was no pus to be drained. And five days later he was leaving the hospital cured not knowing who had cured him, what had cured him, only that he was cured. And his parents were so pleased. The other assistants did not know what it was, the nurse did not know what it was. But my assistant went to the professor and said, "I must tell you, Doctor. I gave him two homoeopathic remedies". And the professor was very intelligent. He said, "If ever I am sick I will take a homoeopathic remedy". (Prolonged applause).

Section 2: The Art of Interrogation

THE ART OF INTERROGATION

In choosing a subject, I have taken as my theme one after which so many beginners are sighing and to which I have, in fact, found really no sufficient and useful references in our homeopathic literature, however extensive.

On the other hand, I have learned through frequenting homeopathic dispensaries and hospitals how very rarely indeed did the practitioners really know how to apply exactly the teachings recommended by the Master, concerning the interrogation of the sick and homeopathic semiology; for, must we, after having listened to the patient, *direct* the interrogation in a given direction, either on the side of a presumed pathological diagnosis or toward a remedy suggested by the first recital made by the patient?

Or must we, against all we were taught in our studies, interrogate without any consideration whatever concerning either remedy or diagnosis, but make what we may call a *systematic* interrogation?

On the other hand, we all know the theoretical principles, but how many *apply* them *really fully?*

Is this question of interrogation simply a thing of theoretical interest or is it a matter of practical application?

Is it only a simple *vue de l'esprit?*

Is there real accord between theory and practice?

Now that homeopathy is developing and growing, and this especially in our Latin countries, France, Switzerland, Spain, Italy and South America, everywhere we hear young practitioners asking: "*But how to question the patient?*", "*What are the most useful and indispensable questions to ask?*", *What is the difference between the allopathic and the homeopathic consultation?*"

Theoretically speaking, we have certainly many precious *practical* suggestions concerning the questionnaire; *Hahnemann,* in his Organon, devotes more than sixty three paragraphs[1] where he speaks about the examination of the patient. *Von Boenninghausen* gives us excellent advice how to take the case. *Jahr* furnishes also a questionnaire, as well as others like *Mure, Perussel, Molinari, Landry, Claude,* then, more

---

1 *§§ concerning the Interrogatoire, in S. Hahnemann's Organon, 5th French edition: 81-104, 139-141, 150-152, 167-171, 175, 177, 179m 181-184, 192, 198-200, 206-21, 216-220, 224, 240, 250, 253-256, 278*

recently, *Close* and *Kent,* this last the only one who gives us a full questionnaire comprising more than thirty-two pages, entitled "What the Doctor Needs to Know in order to Make a Successful Prescrip-tion."

Finally, there is that of *Dr. Margaret Tyler.*

But, I bear in mind also the famous lecture of *Constantine Hering,* published in 1833 in the "Bibliothéque Homeopathique de Genève," in which he sets forth the theme how to trace the picture of the disease, his rules being summed up in four words:-

To listen, to write, to question, to co-ordinate.

It will not be my task this evening to develop theoretically these four precepts, my purpose being essentially to aim at the most useful and exclusively practical side of the question in general.

Consequently, I will not discuss the art of listening to the patient, not the best way to write one's observations, not yet the technique of the study and the co-ordination of the symptoms, or the question of the physical examination. We will take up this evening only with the third precept, the questioning, or examination, strictly speaking.

I will neither enter into long theoretical details about this question, nor propose to you the large ideal questionnaire, which would be the most complete and the most perfect. I have compiled a questionnaire of that kind after years of the study of my chronic cases, but as it covers more than thirty-six pages, I obviously cannot discuss it here.

The main purpose of the *allopathic consultation* is to establish a pathological diagnosis, to label the disease in the most modern nosological fashion. It is said and taught everywhere that without it no treatment should be attempted. For the old school, the investigation of objective pathological symptoms is absolutely essential. In this research, the interrogation plays rather a secondary role, examinations with a more or less complicated array of physical instruments or chemical analysis, but one moment of reflection only will show us that all these procedures only aim at determining the one or the many organs which are affected and to determine how far they are involved.

It is the hunting after end-products, after the results of disease.

If these results are not still manifested in a precise objective manner, and if the sick person suffers from functional troubles only, or even if these are not yet present and the patient is only complaining of subjective troubles, his case is arbitrarily decided. It is a nervous, psychic, imaginary case!

But in the *homeopathic consultation,* we are not at all satisfied with this investigation only. Its object is to establish how a given morbid affection has developed itself in a given subject, and to explore all the possible details of the evolution of such a disease in an individual, and how precisely this patient differs from all the others bearing the same diagnosis.

For example, an allopath, after having examined the throat of a patient, remarks that it is inflamed and covered with membranes from which he may take a part for laboratory examination. And, if the result of this examination be diphtheria, he will give an injection of serum. If it is said to be a simple infection, he will give an antiseptic gargle and a throat-paint.

If he has ten patients following the same diagnosis, the ten will be treated just the same.

(Which reminds me *á propos* of an amusing story a minister told me the other day. He used to wait outside the surgery for a certain doctor friend of his, to whom he ventured to make the remark it was always interesting to note how many of the patients came out with bottles of the same colored medicine. To this remark the only answer forthcoming was a look of rather confused embarrassment!)

On the contrary, a homeopath will inquire into all details which *differentiate* this *particular* patient from the ten others; one would have the membranes on the right side, another on the left, and another on the velum of the palate. The appearance of the membrane may vary in color from green to yellow, black or white, according to the case; in others the consistency may, however, change, but especially interesting for the homeopath are the functional and subjective troubles of the patient. One may have burning or shooting pains, or may complain of dryness or rawness. Certain patients may alleviate their pain by drinking cold water or warm, or by eating solid food. The extension of the trouble from left to right or *vice versa,* or from the throat to the larynx or to the nose, all these differences may lead to a different homeopathic remedy.

Many details, forsooth seemingly of secondary importance, if not quite useless for the allopath, pathologically observed, which will however permit not only of precise diagnosis of the disease but especially the diagnosis of this given patient, and the homeopathic physician will be able to find his *own and particular* remedy, I mean the remedy adapting itself precisely to all the different characteristics and peculiarities of the case.

There exist more than fifty-six remedies for diphtheria, but there is a very small number corresponding really to all the symptoms pertaining to this particular patient. And this is where the task of the homeopath begins.

To know well how to observe, how exactly to interrogate, is the first step in this indispensable inquiry, and one which leads to the real remedy to be found.

This is, Mr. President, ladies and gentlemen, *why* I will take this evening in consideration the best questionnaire which will satisfy the following desiderata:

1. The minimum of the best questions to be asked from a patient when the time is limited.

2. Most important and most necessary those questions to discover, not the pathological diagnosis but the therapeutic diagnosis, the general remedy corresponding to *the patient.*

3. The questions to be asked, those for which we are sure to find a correspondence in our repertories and materia medica.

The interrogation, above all, must be *methodical.*

Of course, it goes without saying that the questions asked must be according to the purest principles of homeopathy, i.e.,

1. *To avoid direct questions,* for we know, if the patient answers with yes or no, the question is badly formed.

2. *Never to ask a question putting an answer, so to say, into the patient's mouth,* thus making sure not to bias his answer.

3. *To avoid all questions where the patient is obliged to choose* between two different alternatives, and respect the sacred rule to leave the patient always his own choice.

Of course, the physician must put himself, as Dr. Kent says, on the level of language comprehended by his patient. His attitude of seriousness and benevolence must help to stimulate the confidence of his patient.

On the other hand, he must know sufficiently his materia medica, so that his questions will be adapted to the comparison he will have to make further on. "Store up your materia medica so as to use it, and it will flow out as your language flows," in the well-known words of Kent.

The physician, by his manner of interrogation and general questions, must do everything not to determine, but to let the patient himself characterize the particular facts. "Say as little as you can, but keep the patient talking and help him to come close to the line and keep to the point."

Never allow yourself to hurry a patient, establish a fixed habit of examination that will stay with you. It is only when you keep up the most careful kind of work that you can set up your reputation and fulfill your highest use (Kent).

We can never sufficiently bear in mind how difficult is the art of interrogation, and all the importance that should be given to it. "One can learn very much from Socrates," observes Hering, "and the study of Plato is as important for us as Hippocrates."

To avoid all ambiguity, I will first give you some questions that in the course of your own practice you also will have frequently heart, demonstrating that many physicians show by the questions they ask that they have not grasped the thought of individualization. For example:

1. Direct questions:

   i. Are you thirsty?

ii. Are you irritable?

iii. Have you got pain in the stomach?

2. Suggestive questions:

i. You do not stand the cold very well, do you?

ii. You surely prefer to be consoled?

iii. I suppose that you don't like too greasy and too rich food?

3. Questions where the patient must choose:

i. Do you prefer dry or wet weather?

ii. Do you dream about sad or cheerful things?

iii. Are your menses dark or light?

About the direct questions, it is quite frequent that a patient would say "Yes, I am thirsty," because he thinks about his morning coffee and his soup at noon but really does not drink anything besides. Or another would say "No," because he thinks that drinking tea, wine, lemon squash and soda do not mean thirst, this being reserved for ordinary water only.

Then, about the greasy or rich food, he will say that he does not like them because the doctor has said, "Too greasy." And about the menses, you will hear that they are dark, being really absolutely red, because a timid patient, having no choice between dark or light, will reply one or the other color in order to get rid of the question.

I think it is unnecessary to discuss every possible answer or error which will result by doing so, my purpose being to give you a list of questions avoiding precisely these errors, to present them to the criterium of your long experience and to submit it to your considered criticism. Of course, you are aware of the considerable advantage a beginner in homeopathy would have if he had not to wait for forty years, but be at once able to ask just the best and most exact questions aiming at a practical result, and to the answer of which he would be able to find a similar correspondence in our pathogenesis.

What would be really the use of a question about which we know no corresponding remedy? Of course, everything is useful, but I repeat that we are working here for practical results and not for theoretical purposes. We must adapt ourselves to the pathogenetic pictures of our materia medica, pictures which are very rich and precious.

To finish with this introduction, I cannot sufficiently criticize the method quoted in the book recently published, "La doctrine de l'Homeopathic francaise" where the physician, after a short physical examination, asks the patient about the symptoms of *Sepia* suggested by a yellow saddle he has observed on her nose, or those of *Lycopodium* on an irritable man complaining of his liver. This we may call the "torpedo method," in French "le torpillage." Because a patient has red lips you would ask him, "Have you got an empty, all-gone sensation in the stomach before noon?" "Do you not find it disagreeable to be in a standing position quite a while?" "Are you not obliged to put your feet out of the bed at night because they are burning." "You probably drink much and eat little, etc. ...."

Those two torpillage methods, the last one based only on direct and suggestive questions, the former one on two external symptoms, are most dangerous, especially for the beginner, as almost invariably a suggestionable patient impressed by the physician, will find present all the symptoms about which he is asked.

One may feel why such physicians do need to give drainage remedies in addition to four or five others, to be able to obtain something we will call a result.

It is *blunderbuss shooting,* ladies and gentlemen, for beginners of course a strong temptation, may be even an amusing method, even perhaps a necessary stage to something better. But the practitioner who is not afraid to work his materia medica, to study his repertories and to understand his Organon, will be able with a single shot—may I say, after the manner of my own fellow-countryman, Wilhelm Tell, "with one arrow"-to obtain the desired results, because his methodical and serious interrogation will give him a full picture of the disease, about which he will be able to consider what represents really the patient on the whole.

I will consider this matter later on.

We have classified our work in the following way:

1. What are the bases of interrogation? (That is, on what basis are the questions to be asked?)

2. What is the best classification to adopt in interrogation?

3. How to formulate the questions, in which way to be formulated?

4. How are we to know if questions are well asked, and consequently well answered?

5. I say again that I will not present here a *full* questionnaire, but the best and shortest questionnaire calculated to obtain the maximum results, the time being limited. And this will constitute the current questionnaire of the physician having at his disposal twenty to thirty minutes for the interrogation and examination of his patient.

WHAT ARE THE BASES OF INTERROGATION?

That is on what basis are the questions to be asked?

To this, I will answer that those questions must be ruled by the homeopathic semiology concerning the value of symptoms, considering always the patient in general, on the whole, to see the patient in his totality and not in his parts; not the disease, not the pathology, not the diagnosis, but the patient, living, feeling and thinking.

Of course, I will not consider the anamnesis, the part concerning hereditary and personal antecedents'; all references which are a part, evidently, of the interrogation of every patient, but not necessary to develop, as they offer absolutely no difficulties to the physician in comparison with the *active interrogation,* after the patient has exposed freely all his feelings and symptoms to his physician. Everyone should be very conversant with the masterly exposition given by Kent in his 23-26 lectures on his homeopathic philosophy.

WHAT CLASSIFICATION IS TO BE ADOPTED?

On one side, we have the counsel given by Hahnemann in his Organon, then the remarkable study of Kent in his 32-33 chapters concerning the value of symptoms, then the numerous classifications established by Grimmer, Gladwin, Green, Loos, Margaret Tyler, Del Mas, Stearns, to quote only those worthy of notice. It is impossible to discuss here every one of the proposed classifications, the broad lines of which, nevertheless, converge in the same direction: First mental symptoms, then general symptoms, then cravings and aversions, then sexual symptoms, including M.P., and finally sleep and dreams.

After this list come the local symptoms related to the organs.

But if, theoretically, this classification seems the most acceptable, practically, it is not so; and about this, experience has proved to me precious teachings.

In my early days of practice, I used always first to ask the mental symptoms, but very soon I came to see I was mistaken.

In fact, an unknown patient, knowing nothing whatever about homeopathy, feels hurt or resents this interrogation about his character when he comes to see you for a headache, a stye or an enlargement of his prostate. Very often too, he imagines that you are mistaking him for a mental case, and that you are making a disguised psychoanalysis. Very shortly, the physician sees by the patient's way of answering, his attitude and his look, the error he himself is committing.

On the other hand, to make the interrogation of the mental symptoms at the end of the questionnaire is also a mistake. Because then the patient is tired and has his mind on the fact that those questions have nothing to do with his disease, and have no relation whatever to it. Thus, he answers shortly, curtly, badly, manifesting very soon his impatience and his desire to get rid of the inquiry.

This is why experience has taught us that it is preferable to begin with the general symptoms, then to ask the questions related to the mentality, explaining rapidly to the patient the difference here between homeopathy and allopathy, the former being able to compare these symptoms with those obtained on the man in health, because of homeopathic experimentation only supposed to be made on the healthy man, and not, as the ordinary school does, on animals.

Then come the aversions and alimentary cravings, then the symptoms related to the sleep and dreams, and finally, for ladies, those concerning the menses, if it is possible to do so. The questions related to the sexual sphere can almost never be asked in the first consultation, especially in a short one. Sometimes it can be touched on when one is asked about heredity or personal history.

To close with, it is good to reconsider some of the symptoms predicated by the patient, especially those considered as rare, peculiar and striking, strange or uncommon, and to examine their modalities in order to see if really they deserve important consideration.

Here is the list of symptoms to be taken into consideration:

General symptoms

Horary aggravation, periodical season aggravation; by the weather; dry, wet, cold, hot, fog, sun, wind. Changes of weather: snow, storms; aggravation of temperature, draughts of air; tendency to take cold, desire or aggravation by the air; aggravation of position, by motion or by repose, riding in cars, sailing, prandial aggravation, appetite and thirst, aggravation by certain foods, wine, tobacco, drugs, vaccinations, cold or hot baths, seashore or mountain, clothing, wounds slow to heal, hemorrhages, fainting in rooms full of people, laterality (side affected).

Mental symptoms

The mental state of a human being can, on the whole, be resolved into four or five essential points; life or death, emotions, fears, irritability and sadness; and all these under hyper or hypo-manifestations.

The theoretical classification would be thus:

1. Symptoms relating to the instinct of self-preservation (death, suicide, etc.).
2. Ailments from grief, vexation, mortification, indignation, anger, bad news, disappointed love, etc.
3. Fear, anguish, anxiety.
4. Irritability, anger, violence, impatience, hastiness.
5. Sadness, weeping, despair, effect of consolation.

Then, certain symptoms having no relation to these categories as, for example, jealousy, absent-mindedness, concentration, mania of scrupules and as to trifles; modifications of the character before, during and after menses.

Instead of following this questionnaire in the above given order, it would be better to follow it in the reverse order; because one must begin with symptoms rather superficial and which do not go too deep into the mind of the patient, which latter is ultimately to be discovered.

For the practitioner who has his eyes open as well as his understanding, there are numerous mental symptoms that can be observed without saying one single word, as for example; timidity, loquacity, egotism, easily offended, embarrassed, exhilarated, easily startled, haughty, needless, suspicious, laughing immoderately, even some memory troubles, quiet or hurrying disposition, sighing patients, restless, weeping when speaking about certain symptoms; also, there are certain symptoms of which there is no need to ask the patient because he will tell them himself, either because he came for this purpose, or suffers really very much on account of it. Very often, also, friends or relatives may have written of those symptoms to you before the consultation, if they are sufficiently striking, as, for example, the refusal to eat, the desire to escape, sometimes even fear of suicide, etc.

Aversions and Alimentary Cravings

i. Sweets, pastry, delicacies.

ii. Salty things.

iii. Sour, strong and spiced food.

iv. Greasy and rich foods, butter.

v. Bread, fruits, fish, meat.

vi. Milk, coffee, wine, beer.

vii. State of thirst and appetite.

Sleep and Dreams

i. Position of the body, head and extremities during sleep.

ii. What the patient is doing during sleep; laughs, starts, talks, shrieks, weeps, is afraid, grinds his teeth, keeps eyes or mouth open, etc.

iii. Quality of the sleep: hours and causes of waking, of sleeplessness and sleepiness.

iv. All about dreams.

Symptoms concerning the menses and the sexual sphere

i. M.P. too late, duration, abundance, color, quality, consistence, more day or night, influence of the character or other particular symptoms before, during and after the M.P., shortly all about what we call the "Molimen."

Rare, strange and peculiar symptoms

Uncommon symptoms indicated by the patient, with their modalities and related phenomena and the making more precise of the main symptoms for which the consultation was made.

Now, let us see this theoretical list of questions realized in a practical way, according to the Hahnemannian principles. I have just purposely chosen questions corresponding to repertory rubrics, which are of a middle size and containing, when possible, two or three degrees of remedies (italic and heavy type) and avoided the longer paragraphs like those of sadness, night aggravation, thirst, etc., which contain almost all the remedies.

HOW TO FORMULATE THE QUESTIONS

It is not a bad procedure to say to the patient at this time: "I have listened to you until now without interrupting you, now we will change the role, and please don't be astonished if I seemingly stop you while answering, to ask you the next question, because this will mean that the answer I was waiting for is obtained. Do not believe that by so doing, I under-estimate your answer, but this only signifies that a longer explanation will bring neither useful nor new details in the case."

General Symptom

1. At what time in the twenty-four hours do you feel worst?
2. In which season do you feel less well?
3. How do you stand the cold, hot, dry, wet weather?
4. How does fog affect you?
5. What do you feel when exposed to the sun?

6. How does change of weather affect you?

7. What about snow?

8. What kind of climate is objectionable to you, and where would you choose to spend your vacation?

9. How do you feel before, during and after a storm?

10. What are your reactions to north wind, south wind, to the wind in general?

11. What about draughts of air and changes of temperature?

12. What about warmth in general, warmth of the bed, of the room, of the stove?

13. How do you react to extremes of temperature?

14. What difference do you make in your clothing in winter?

15. What about taking colds in winter and in other seasons?

16. How do you keep your window at night?

17. What position do you like best—sitting, standing, lying?

18. How do you feel standing a while, or kneeling in church?

You remark that this question of the standing position comes again. You will find this way of repeating it is intentional here and there in the questionnaire. It is a very useful and necessary procedure for verification.

19. What sports do you engage in?

20. What about riding in cars or sailing?

21. How do you feel before, during and after meals?

22. What about your appetite, how do you feel if you go without a meal?

    It will be often answered to you: "I can easily go without a meal but I never can stand a big dinner or banquet." A question that you did not ask, but which demonstrates that the question was well formulated as it made the patient talk and left him his own choice.

23. What quantity and what do you drink? What about thirst?

24. What are the foods that make you sick, and why?

    (If the patient does not answer after a while, just ask looking closely at him: sweets, salty things, sour, greasy food, eggs, meat, pork, bread, butter, vegetables, cabbages, onions, fruits?)

25. What about wine, beer, coffee, tea, milk, vinegar?

26. How much do you smoke in a day, and how do you feel after smoking?

27. What are the drugs to which you are very sensitive or which make you sick?

28. What are the vaccinations you have had, and the results from them?

29. What about cold or warm baths, sea baths?

30. How do you feel at the seaside, or on high mountains?

31. How do collars, belts and tight clothing affect you?

32. How long are your wounds in healing, how long in bleeding?

33. In what circumstances have you felt like fainting.

Mental Symptoms

34. What are the greatest griefs that you have gone through in your life?

    (Quite often the patient will lower the head and look quite moved, and a kind word of the doctor will be needed. It is why, as soon as the extra-version or self-expression has been made, this following question will make the patient look at you again in an astonished way, and sometimes with a happy smile).

35. What are the greatest joys you have had in life?

    These two questions are very important and, when asked at the right moment, will pave the way for the coming questions.

36. At what time in the twenty-four hours do you feel in the blues, depressed, sad, pessimistic?

37. How do you stand worries?

38. On what occasions do you weep?

(If the patient cannot answer, we will just ask – not losing for one second his expression – music, at reproaches, at which time of the day? Certain people can refrain from weeping, some others cannot).

39. What effect has consolation on you?

(If the answer is, "It depends by whom," you may say; "just by people you like," because very often people say they do not like to be comforted because they think of members of their family they hate.)

40. On what occasions do you feel despair?

41. In what circumstances have you ever felt jealous?

42. When and on what occasions do you feel frightened or anxious?

(If the patient does not answer, ask, some people are afraid of the night, of darkness, to be alone, of robbers, of certain animals, of death, of certain diseases, of ghosts, to lose their reason, of noises at night, of poverty, of storm, of water. According to the way of answering, you will at once see the real fears, and be able to discriminate those which are not to be taken into consideration.)

43. How do you feel in a room full of people, at church, at a lecture?

44. Do you go red or white when you are angry, and how do you feel afterwards?

45. How do you stand waiting?

    (If he does not answer, just question him about impatience.)

46. How rapidly do you walk, eat, talk, write?

47. What have been the complaints or effects following chagrin, grief, disappointed love, vexation, mortification, indignation, bad news, fright?

48. In time of depression, how do you look at death?

    (Certain patients have presentiments of death, thoughts of death, even desire to die; others have tendencies or desires of suicide, some would be courageous enough to do it, others are afraid, in spite of desiring it.)

49. Tell me all about over-conscientiousness and over scrupulousness, about trifles; some people do not care about too much details and too much order.

50. What about your character before, during and after menses?

During all these questions, the physician must by kind words put his patient at ease, but must watch him very closely, without the patient's noticing it.

Food Cravings and Aversions

1. What is the kind of food for which you have a marked craving or aversion, or what are those that make you sick or you cannot eat?

   Here also, it is very important to watch very carefully the expression of the patient, because it is very easy to read on the face by observing the corners of the mouth coming down if the patient is disgusted, or on the contrary coming up with big shining eyes if the craving or a strong alimentary attraction is felt. Then, one can add, for example:

2. What about pastry and sweets?

3. What about sour or spiced food?

4. What about rich or greasy food?

5. How much salt do you need for your taste?

6. What about thirst and what do you drink?

   Coffee, wine, beer, etc...

   Of course, all those questions have been already asked in the beginning of the questionnaire, but by asking them again, you are able, by doing some cross questioning, to determine if they have been answered well the first time or not.

Sleep

1. In which position do you sleep, and since when that position? Where do you put your arms, and how do you like to have your head?

2. What are you doing during sleep?

   (If the patient does not answer, you add, some people speak, laugh, shriek, weep, are restless, and are afraid, grind their teeth, have their mouth or their eyes open.)

3. At what time do you wake up, or when are you sleepy? What makes you restless or sleepy?

4. What about dreams?

For Ladies - Menses

1. At what age did they begin?

2. How frequently do they come?

3. What about their duration, abundance, color, odor, what about clots, etc.

4. At what time in the twenty-four hours do they flow most?

5. How do you feel before, during and after menses?

Retaking the Case

It is necessary to take through again in the symptoms told by the patient, those which were strange, rare and peculiar, for example, sensation of a nail in the head; feeling of a string drawing back the eyeballs, feeling of a lump in the throat, a griping feeling in the heart, feeling of a constriction like a bandage around the knees.

All those must be carefully noted, in order that the physician may ascertain himself that there are no occasional causes provoking them.

Then, about some other outstanding symptoms; it is important to take the modalities concerning the aggravation or amelioration by motion, repose, heat or cold, in or outdoors, position, eating, pressure, etc.

HOW NOW, TO KNOW IF THE QUESTIONS ARE WELL ASKED AND, CONSEQUENTLY, WELL ANSWERED?

There are two ways of knowing:

1. During all the interrogation, the physician must carefully watch his patient and observe the way he answers. As in La Fontaine's fable, the "rampage" must accord with the "plumage," i.e., the intonation of his voice, the play and expression of his physiognomy, especially in mouth and eyes, must be carefully observed and grasped.

   A patient who says, "Yes, I like meat, but I don't drink milk with pleasure" without change of expression indicates no symptom at all. But if he says, "Oh, I cannot do without meat, and I hate milk," saying this with a happy face and an enlargement of the eyes regarding meat, but regarding milk with a wry face, while turning the head to the side, you then know you have good symptoms.

Of course, beside the question of useful and useless symptoms, in the useful symptoms there is still a gradation. There are very marked and also less important ones, but this comes into consideration only if we have quite a number of them. On the occasion of the first interrogation, we will have little to do with this consideration, and be happy to have only a sufficient number of symptoms.

2. During the interrogation, the physician is carefully noting in writing all the answers of his patient. He underlines or marks with a cross those which are of importance to be further cross-questioned or verified in order to be assured that the patient has *really well understood and well answered* the question.

   This is to put it to the proof.

Then, we have seriously to consider making quite a number of cross-questions. For example:

If the patient has told you that he feels worse after meals, you may ask him, "If you have an important matter to decide or a delicate letter to write, or some important call to make, would you do it at 2 p.m.?"

If he told you that he was sleeping with his hands outstretched over his head, you may ask him, "During sleep, would the warmth of the bed clothes cause your hands to perspire?"

If he tells you that he hates greasy food, "Do you prefer the fish with sauce, or fried, or in black butter? And how do you like bacon?"

If he says that pity or consolation aggravate him, ask him if he has a friend to whom he gives his confidence when he is worried.

Should he assert he is never angry, ask him if he is red or white when angry. Very often, the answer will be, "Red, but it passes rapidly away."

To be certain that some symptoms are to be retained and good, these few above-mentioned examples will suggest you to know how to ask these questions.

Very often, a patient says that he is very impatient, but you can observe that, after having sat for half an hour in your waiting room, he walks calmly into your consulting room and responds most calmly to your questions.

Another will tell you that he is even-tempered, but you learn that he is divorced or that he has left his family because of incompatibility of character.

If one, two or more remedies come to your mind after such an examination, and you are hesitating between this one and the other, that is the only occasion where one is authorized to ask some questions, always based on the same principles, but relative to the symptoms characteristic of the remedy suggested, always, obviously trying to avoid direct questions and the torpillage methods already referred to. Very often, it would be better and more prudent to give S.L., rather than to administer a remedy that is not absolutely indicated, about which we are not sure, and have the courage to await the second consultation in order to complete the picture of the disease.

The purpose of this paper is not to examine what is to be done with the symptoms thus obtained or how to classify them, or how to find the corresponding simillimum in the materia medica. If one follows this classification, the second part of the work, the grading and classification of symptoms would be nearly completed for the physician.

I observed that certain questions are always answered in the same way, by almost everybody, and consequently I consider those bad questions. Sometimes, too, the patient indicates some symptoms which seems very important, and which he has not in reality. He will inform you that he has some abilities or qualities, and you observe just the contrary.

That is why I think that a questionnaire established with method and reflection is indispensable, and that is why I have submitted it to you this evening, desiring to know your own experiences and what are the questions to suppress, to develop, or in which order to ask them.

I always try to practice the advice of my esteemed teacher, Dr. Austin of New York, who told me that a good physician should be able in the first consultation to make his patient laugh or cry, and so doing, he was assured that the contact was made, as he was able to put in vibration the living human being who was asking for *help*.

If, in the allopathic consultation, as we were told and taught in our allopathic studies, one must not believe his patient, must ask the fewest questions possible and believe only what could be observed by the physician himself, this is quite different in homeopathic consultation, because the homeopathic physician must do his best to create around him an atmosphere of confidence and benevolence, and try to comprehend especially the human being who comes to be helped. The most important task in homeopathy is to individualize and to discriminate, but individualization and comparison are inseparable, and there is a difference in the nature of things most similar, a point that must be carefully considered.

The substitution of one remedy for another cannot be thought of or entertained in homeopathy, and Kent repeats what Hahnemann says: "In homeopathy, medicines can never replace each other nor be as good as another."

One cannot repeat enough that if the first examination is well established, well made, well realized and well interpreted, the search after the remedy will be but a sole thing, and if the case has been well taken and the remedy based really on the most important symptoms, all this being rightly done at the first consultation, the work for the physician will be considerably easier because he has found the thread and has only to follow it. On the contrary, this treatment based on local examination or insufficient interrogation will oblige you to zigzag perpetually and, instead of feeling your prescription based on an edifice with large foundations, you have the impression of a cork floating on the ocean.

Nothing is more culpable than to say, "*Thuja* is your remedy, because I see that you are perspiring on your upper lip!" (the repertory has seven remedies for this sole symptom) or, "You are *Lachesis* because your lips are blue and varnished," or "You are a case of *Condurango* because you have cracks in the corners of the mouth."

If I speak here about *Condurango*, it is to confess my *mea culpa*.

Eleven years ago, when I came to the London Homeopathic Hospital for the first time, I was very kindly authorized to follow the visiting physician round the wards. It happened to be the day of Sir J. Weir. I did not know him; was he a good or a bad homeopath? Did he know anything about it? Very soon I would be able to decide for myself.

Just arrived from Geneva, after having studied homeopathy in the "Catechism of Dr. Dewey" and the "Organon of Hahnemann," I thought I had the whole of homeopathic knowledge and wisdom. This was all the more so as I had already treated some cases with success, having received the benefit of the experience of a physician who had given me advice in some rather more difficult cases.

After having seen some patients, we stopped before a bed where a new patient had just come, and I still remember and can see Sir John Weir, his head bending towards the patient, asking innumerable questions. As soon as one was answered, another was quickly formulated.

In the beginning, this impressed me, but I rapidly saw that the patient had quite a red patch on the right corner of her mouth with a deep crack.

This reminded me of a similar case where I was puzzled about the indicated remedy and where a homeopath told me: "It is a plain *Condurango* case." As soon as Sir John Weir was through, feeling the marked superiority of my knowledge and seeing that after this long and elaborate interrogation he had not mentioned any remedy, I told him, "Don't you see that it is a plain case of *Condurango*?" Very kindly he turned his head and, without irony or reproach but bowing his head, he said very politely: "I thank you, Sir; we will discuss this later on." Everyone around turned on me with an appreciative look at my cleverness.

After the visit we went down, and I then had my bad quarter of an hour *(mauvais quart d'heure)* – my cold douche.

"Well," said Sir John, "why is it a case of *Condurango*? Simply because of this crack in the corners of the mouth." "But," said he, "what about all her other symptoms?"

"Oh, they are of no importance. If you look carefully at her tongue, you surely will find some denuded areas and also some gastric symptoms and this will confirm and prove your *Condurango*."

"Well, well," said Sir John, "let us see." He simply opened a large book like the Bible and asked me if I knew it. "No." said I; "have homeopaths written such large books?" "It is the Repertory of Kent," he replied, "and see here that twenty-two remedies stand beside *Condurango* for cracks in the mouth."

With kindness but persuasion he very rapidly pulled to pieces all my illusions and my assurance.

He convinced me that this was a case of *Sepia*, explaining to me patiently why among the many symptoms there was a discrimination to be made, how interesting and of the utmost importance a hierarchic classification was to be made and that rules and principles were to be followed for such a study, why *Sepia* was the remedy for this patient and not *Condurango*. It was the most beautiful lesson in modesty that I ever received.

I shriveled inside and perspired outside. I had brilliantly demonstrated my deep and profound ignorance and unveiled my incapacity. But I probably was still not baptized, as when I went to New York, Dr. Austin at my first interview asked me which were the homeopathic remedies for rheumatism and, after I had spoken about *Rhus-tox.* and *Bryonia,* he gave me the last blow to my knowledge, saying simply:

"Well, my brother, I think it will be necessary to study homeopathy."

Thus, I learned to live out this famous sentence of the philosopher: "All I know is, that I know, I know nothing!"

In the same way, if your interrogation is not based on the essential principles of the homeopathic doctrine, if you are led by your caprice or fancy only and interrogate just about the symptoms the patient is complaining of, you will make only patchwork and end in failure. This failure would only demonstrate your own ignorance.

If a patient presents herself to you with varicose veins and pain in the lower limbs and you give her *Fluoric acid, Calcarea fluorica* or *Hamamelis,* you will have treated only the vascular walls, but not all the varicose patient. This is only a travesty of homeopathy. It is the application of a remedy to a diagnosis, it is allopathic prescribing with homeopathic remedies.

If the patient adds that she has agglutinated eyes in the morning and that her hairs are falling away, you would think at once of *Graphites* or *Sulphur.* But if she adds still further that she is bleeding from the nose, is very thirsty and craving acids, you will turn your preference to *Phosphorus.* You may then ask if she feels an empty sensation at the stomach and suffers from heartburn, in consultation, she will confess that she is suffering from a very distended abdomen, that she is constipated, her sleep is unrefreshing, liking better to be outdoors, so you will say: "Now it is clear, it is *Lycopodium*," and so on, continually. Like the wandering Jew, you err in this labyrinth, losing your head and often your patience. Why? Because you have not made a systematic and methodical examination, established according to the rules formerly given.

If you go through the short, but quite full interrogation given before, you will learn that this patient has her menses more at night, and the study of this case will show you very rapidly and clear as water that only one remedy covers all these symptoms, except the varicose veins, it is true, and here the remedy is *Magnesia carbonica*, not for or against the varicose veins, but *for* the patient who will be cured, and the varicose veins besides.

I described this case *en passant* because it is precisely one of my successful cures of varicose veins. The patient was cured, her varicose veins disappeared, like all the other miseries: gastritis, epistaxis, etc.... You will not be astonished to know that this depressed patient is now cheerful and enterprising, and that the beautiful mass of her black hair justifies her legitimate pride.

The homeopathic interrogatory includes, as you see, rules to be followed and a technique to be observed.

This interrogation, made according to the suggestions given in the beginning of this paper, will permit of the physician individualizing his case after an interrogation well made, a precious stone in the walls of the therapeutic edifice.

Physicians cannot sufficiently avoid every partiality to influence the patient from whom he has to elicit symptoms, related to remedies of which he may think, and which come to his mind by the first answer given by the patient. "He has a key to the patient and examines the patient by the key, that is, as Kent says, by the drug, a bad practice and never to be resorted to except as a dernier resort and in stupid patient." Doing so, we are on the wrong track which will end only in pitfalls.

The more objective the symptoms, the more they are to be observed of the patient dead, in his coffin, the less value have they. On the contrary, the more they express the living, feeling, thinking human being, the more important they are.

To establish a questionnaire really useful to the busy physician for his daily practice, a questionnaire based on the pure doctrine of homeopathy, such has been my purpose this evening. My endeavour will be more than fully rewarded and compensated if I may be told what further to add, to take away, to modify or to render it more perfect.

Knowing the valued knowledge and opinions of the members of your society, I submit this most important question to your esteemed consideration.

The Homeopathic Recorder.

PHARMACOPOLLAXY

This term is derived from the union of two Greek words *Pharmacon*, meaning remedy, and *pollaxis*, meaning many times, and means really, *'the repetition of the remedy.'*

It is not my purpose to develop here all the modalities concerning this controversed question, which has been also applied so differently, but to place myself to a higher point of view, and here I will put the question in those terms: What do we mean by the repetition of the remedy?

At first, it seems that this question is very simple and clear, nevertheless it has been so much obscured that one could find commonly in our school this too frequently used expression: *the repetition of the dose.* What signifies this locution? Dr. Jahr asserts that the administration of the remedy in watery solution does not constitute a repetition, of the dose. This is really the way to darken and complicate this subject. No, the fact of giving a remedy in a successive manner, no matter in which form, is not – homeopathically speaking—a fraction of this remedy, but really the repetition of the very remedy each time it is given.

This is why Hahnemann, in his first volume of the Materia Medica, in the French edition, stipulates in his eighth paragraph this very question, writing as the title of his chapter:

On the repetition of homeopathic medicaments.

The master could have said in this title: the repetition of the doses, if it had been his opinion. So, it seems clear that in his very thoughts, every time one is repeating a dose he is repeating the remedy and the *whole remedy.* This chapter begins with those words:

"In the Organon I have insisted on the necessity never to give at the same time but one single dose of a well chosen homeopathic medicament, and to let it have all the necessary time to develop its action."

Evidently here the words *single dose* signify a remedy given at one single time. Of course, if one repeats many times this dose, he repeats as frequently this remedy.

One gives each time what represents the whole of the remedy, and not a fraction of it. Moreover in the chronic diseases, when we repeat the "dose at long intervals, do we not give each time the remedy?

A little further in this chapter, Hahnemann says again:

"Thus, a primitive psoric eruption, on a patient which is not too much weakened, even if it has invaded the whole body, can be perfectly cured through one dose of Tincture Sulph. Xe (30th dil.) repeated every seven days in the course of ten to twelve weeks" (consequently with 10 to 12 globules).

This term *consequently,* in this parenthesis explains the thought of the master. Those who know and understand the writings of Hahnemann, know very well that for him each globule contains the remedy on the whole.

Here are again some very intelligible and explicit words about it:

"But if the physician has to give a same substance more than one time, what is indispensable in order to cure serious chronic diseases, he should be careful to change each time the degree of dynamization, even very slightly, the vital force of the patient can support the same medicament even at short intervals an incredible number of times, one after another and this with the greatest success..."

Dr. Mure, in his *Doctrine of Rio,* is still clearer and more precise:

"One single globule dissolved in a glass of water and taken by spoonfuls, every twelve hours, constitutes as many doses as the number of spoonfuls taken."

In homeopathy nothing will increase the energy or intensity and the rapidity of actions of remedy by augmenting or multiplying its quantity.

At last, the spirit of our doctrine teaches us that in the series of potentization, each vial contains the remedy on the whole, and every one of the hundred drops of the vial contains the whole remedy, to this degree in the series.

We must never forget, as has been said already by Granier, a French homeopath, that our remedies are not the so-called infinitely smalls, and we must forever let this faulty locution disappear. Our remedies are dynamic agents, like the miasms, and ought to be called *miasmoid*. The presence of matter is here absolutely out of the question.

The doctrine of the repetition of the remedy is virtually contained in the following sentence taken from the writings of our master:

"It goes without saying that before the physician permits himself to repeat the dose of a medicament, he should be absolutely convinced that it was perfectly well chosen and homeopathically indicated."

One should never say *repetition of the dose,* but we should say, *repetition of the remedy*.

Every time Hahnemann speaks about the repetition of the doses, it is only a negligence of language, also every time he speaks of a *medicament* instead of a remedy. In fact, the medicament, through experimentation or proving produces the phenomena and pertains to pathology. The *remedy* on the contrary, through experiments, neutralizes the symptoms and pertains to nosology. To the old school, the remedy is a remedy *a priori,* without anything prior to it, but for our school, the remedy is considered as such only *a posteriori,* having as its starting point its study on the healthy man. To the homeopathic school, every remedy before its application must have been a medicament.

Of course, it is not our purpose on this occasion to give all the wise advices resulting from the vast experience of the master concerning the repetition of the remedy. For those who have taken the time to read carefully and to study the preface of the *Chronic Diseases,* the *Lesser Writings,* the preface of each volume of the *Materia Medica Pura* and the *Organon,* it is very clear to understand that our master has said almost everything touching the pharmacopollaxy.

In conclusion, we can say that:

1. The ideal to be realized, as Hahnemann said, would be to treat every disease with *one single remedy* and one single dose. Of course, this supposes a very careful study and quite perfect correspondence of the remedy to the sick patient.

2. The repetition of the remedy requires positive and strong reasons. The principal reason of the repetition of the remedy must be based on the vital reception, on the individual reaction which is called

susceptibility of the patient, the less sensitive is the patient, the more one is permitted to repeat.

3. The repetition of the remedy depends also on the nature of the remedy.

4. The repetition of the remedy must be submitted to the nature of the disease as well as to the nature of the remedy.

5. The repetition of the remedy depends on the duration of the action of the remedy. Everyone knows that *Calcarea* has a longer duration of action than *Ignatia*.

6. The repetition of the remedy depends on its dynamization (potency).

7. In chronic diseases, one must be very careful with the repetition and you will never regret to repeat at long intervals, rather than too shortly.

8. In acute diseases, experience teaches us that the repetition can be done most frequently. Nevertheless many beautiful cases have been cured with one single dose or a few doses. (High fever, great pain, great fear, strong fits of anger or emotional excitement shorten the action of a remedy and indicate repetition.)

9. Hahnemann has repeated:

"And nothing is more guilty than to repeat blindly and routinarily a remedy, one must be

*guided always by the reaction of the patient and observe carefully the direction and course of the symptoms,... One must be very careful not to use prevision in the indications of the homeopathic remedies and should always base his prescription on the actual totality: it is impossible to prescribe different remedies in advance, either mixed or alternated, for this is a practice absolutely aside from the principles of our doctrine, it is only empiricism, and the work of the most pitiful routine. ... The homeopathic physician ought to examine the symptoms every time he prescribes; otherwise he cannot know whether the same remedy is indicated a second time, or whether a medicine is at all appropriate."**

10. The most important thing about the repetition is the careful observation of the patient and disease, so as to ascertain precisely which is which, pertains to the one or the other. More harm has been done by repeating doses than by giving too rarely a remedy. One is amazed to observe all the possibilities of the single dose when the field for its action is free and no interference perturbs it possibilities. There are great forces that we still do not dream of, and one impulse, as small as it seems to be, has its place in the right moment, according to the law of nature, and can bring results which are really extraordinary.

---

* *Hahnemann, Chronic Diseases, p. 160, loc. cit.*

11. We must add, as Hahnemann says; *There are exceptions to the rule, which it is, however, not the business of every beginner to discover.*

12. The repetition of the remedy is one of the most important things after the careful selection of the remedy and its careful prescription. It needs not a worried, nervous or restless physician; but very careful observation, patience, knowledge and also courage are the qualities required for a master in prescribing. The homeopathic physician is surely the one who must be most careful about this question and who is able to learn very much if he knows how to watch and wait, after having given his remedy. No routine must preside to the decision of such a homeopathician, for he must act only according to law and principles, as Kent beautifully describes it in his chapter concerning the second prescription:

*"No repetition is to be considered unless the record has been again fully studied, unless the first examination, and all the things that have since arisen, have been carefully restudied that they may be brought again to the mind of the physician."**

The Homeopathic Recorder.

---

* *Chronic Diseases, trad. Hempel, 1845, Vol. I, p. 161.*

Section 3: The Hidden Treasures of the Last Organon

THE HIDDEN TREASURES OF THE LAST ORGANON

INNOVATIONS AND LAST ADVICE OF HAHNEMANN

(The British Homoeopathic Journal, July-Oct 1954)

The main points which I wish to raise here are either entirely new or somewhat revolutionary when compared with accepted notions divulged and applied in the five earlier editions of the *Organon,* or points already stated but re-drafted and re-examined. They are, as a rule, badly known or not known at all by Homoeopaths. I shall therefore endeavour to extract them as gold and diamonds are extracted from a mine, and let them sparkle in the sunshine of truth. This is what I propose to do for the benefit of my illustrious colleagues assembled here. I shall not proceed paragraph by paragraph, but by order of importance.

The paragraphs I shall consider first are those of practical interest, and, afterwards, I shall take such para-graphs as are interesting from a theoretical point of view.

1. **PHARMACOPOLLAXY**, or medicamental repetition is, undoubtedly, a question of great interest to all medical men, but it is more particularly so for Homoeopaths who are more especially trained to observe individual reactions. The paragraphs contained in the *Organon* on this subject are the outcome of numerous experiments repeated in the course of Hahnemann's professional activity, that is, over 50 years' practical experience.

   In § 246, he repeats the statement included in the five earlier editions namely, that:

   "Any clearly defined improvement showing obvious progress is a state in which — as long as it lasts —the repeated administration of any medicine whatsoever is to be strictly forbidden, as the remedy previously taken by the patient is still producing its beneficial effect and", Hahnemann adds, "this is no rare occurrence in acute disorders."

Such is the well known and much-quoted paragraph which Hahnemann's and Kent's disciples observe most reverently and to which they owe such excellent results. The words "This is a no rare occurrence...", however, remind me that, though this is fairly frequent, there are a good many cases in which no progress is detected and where it will be necessary to repeat. We shall see later on how this is to be done, but we must bear in mind that Hahnemann never says anything which has not been duly considered and thought out, and that all his words should be weighed with the utmost care. He goes on to say:

"On the other hand, **in chronic disorders which have not reached an advanced stage"!**

mark the words "not reached an advanced stage"!

"the improvement may last from 40 to 60 or even 100 days. This is, however, very rare, and besides, it is important for both physician and patient **to reduce the period in order to effect a speedier cure.** This may be achieved provided the following conditions are observed:

(1) "The choice of the remedy shall be strictly determined in accordance with the Law of Similars.

(2) "It shall be administered in an infinitesimal potency." (I insist upon "dynamization" as the word "dose" implies quantity, whereas dynamization refers to quality).

(3) "After being extensively diluted and highly dynamized.

(4) "Absorbed dissolved in water

(5) "Administered in general in very small quantities (1 coffee-spoonful).

(6) "Repeated at intervals which experience has proved suitable to affect as speedy a cure as possible.

(7) "**Taking great care,** however, in repeating, **to vary the degree of potency so that dose should differ slightly** from those preceding and following."

Where he is at variance with the notions hitherto accepted is in the following recommendations:

i. The absorption of **any homoeopathic remedy to be repeated shall henceforth be exclusively in liquid form.** A new factor in the preparation of remedies is the suppression of attenuations from mother tinctures. All remedies, to whichever natural kingdom they may belong, whether derived from mother tinctures or substance solutions, **must undergo the three traditional centesimal triturations.** Hahnemann **rejects** granules, tablets and triturations (§ 246).

ii. **In acute cases,** where no improvement is observed, the dose is to be repeated and—this is quite new—in chronic diseases where the treatment has proved effective, **the remedy in order to speed up the cure, may be given daily** and for months, if necessary.

In paragraph 247, Hahnemann stresses the danger of repeating the remedy with the same degree of potency, which he defines as: —

> **"inopportune and unwarranted repetition of an unmodified dose** is liable to provoke an absolutely unnecessary morbid addition".

It is detrimental to the patient (§ 247a) to repeat the same remedy on the plea that it has done him good in globules with the same dynamization.

It is also detrimental to the patient if repeated because it has done him good in **liquid** form with the same dynamization.

It is detrimental, too, if repeated with the same attenuation, even if the original preparation has been shaken on each occasion, 10 times, or only twice, because the remedy newly administered is unchanged as regards potency and liable to occasion what is known as **therapeutic saturation.**

In fact, after the first dose of a medicine which has proved efficacious, the patient will be a little less ill. The 2nd dose must consequently be adapted to a less morbid condition, or rather to disease in a more dynamized stage. The patient has been saturated in the first stage, thanks to a remedy in a suitable dose. Consequently Hahnemann recommends giving the same remedy, but more highly dynamized, the disease having been partially **subdued under its influence.**

The remedy is thus to be administered **in varying forms** as the cure proceeds, so as to be constantly adapted to the disease.

Hahnemann combines two factors in an entirely new form. Apparently the remedy was to be given in diluted and dynamized form only, but a notion of quantity was added in order that no confusion should arise as to the notions of **dosing, frequency and dynamization.**

Dosage implies capacity: 1, 2, 3 small, middle-sized or large spoonfuls, i.e., notion of **quantity.**

Frequency is implied by repetition of the dose once, twice, three times. . . .

Dynamization produced by shaking the dilution a certain number of times, implies quality.

Hahnemann now defines quantity (§ 275, 281), i.e., posology, even with high potency, in the form of a single globule of poppy seed size (§ 270f, 272, 279).

PHARMACOPOLLAXY MUST BE ASCENDENCY

For the first time in professional life, Hahnemann lays stress upon the importance of increasing the rate of potency in repeating the dose of a remedy. This had not yet been mentioned in former editions. It is contained in the footnote to § 246 as well as in 248, 270f, 280 and 281, and worded as follows:

> "The remedy is to be administered at a low rate of potency, proceeding according to the technique and after exhaustion of the solution, repeating at a higher rate of power."

Finally, he insists upon the

"danger of repeating with the same potency,

even only once, this being detrimental and even liable to lead to incurability. It is even more harmful that it would be with an equal dose of an Allopathic remedy, as such repetition, through un-warranted dosage, might bring about chronic medicamental dyscrasia, a kind of medicamental miasma, 'This", he adds, "may also occur when the dosage is too high", i.e., when a mouthful or tablespoonful is given instead of a teaspoonful. (In this connection, see § 276 and foot-note to § 282).

I shall not comment on the results of this new prac-tice, nor compare it with Kent's ascendent pharma-copollaxy as it would lead me too far.

However, there is a **very important exception** to which I wish to call your attention in the footnote to § 282, with regard to the doses **in the treatment of the**

three great diatheses during the period of their first cutaneous manifestations, namely:

> **for psora: recent scabieic dermatosis**
>
> **for syphilis: untreated primary canker, wherever located, and**
>
> **for sycosis: condylomata**
>
> **"These localized diseases"** (and not local, I insist upon it) **"do not only tolerate, but demand immediate administration of large doses** (large tablespoonfuls or even mouthfuls) **repeated daily or even several times a day, of their specific remedies in ascending repetition.** In chronic ill-nesses, the doses should at first be as small as possible (a teaspoonful only)".

The volume of the remedy, i.e., the quantity, accord-ing to Hahnemann's experience, must therefore be taken into account.

> **"In such cases particularly,** no objective localization should be suppressed and nothing ought to be removed bv external applications, for **the disappearance of such objective manifestations, which the physician cannot fail to notice, enable him to ascertain that the remedy hitherto administered is no longer necessary."**
>
> Hahnemann adds, however, that

"experience has shown that itch, like syphilitic canker can and must be treated only exceptionally through external channels, but that in the case of sycotic condylomata, internal administration combined with simultaneous external application in direct contact with lesions may prove necessary."

(Footnote to § 282) as the homoeopath never tries to decieve patients by purely superficial success which, though it may be gratifying at first, is always harmful in the long run.

2. **PHARMACOPRAXY**, i.e., the preparation of remedies (§ 264 to 272). Here Hahnemann expounds his absolutely new theory for the preparation of the 50 millesimals as well as the technique of their application. I had, in fact, already read years ago in the BJH, an article on the "plus method". I had even applied it ... and it had been a dead failure. Since then, none of our papers have ever mentioned it. It showed, however, how important it was to have the *Organon* translated, as no one had ever applied the method in the proper way. Even today, I occasionally read in homoeopathic journals about cures affected by 50 millesimals in globules. This is positive proof that the prescribers of such doses have not understood the new method at all, as the remedies ought to be administered **in liquid form only** (§ 271).

In practice the patient is given a capsule containing a single poppy seed size globule crushed in a little sugar of milk. He is instructed to let it dissolve only before taking it. After putting it into a bottle with about 100 grammes of clean and slightly alcoholized water and vigorously shaking it 10 times, he is then to take about a coffee-spoonful morning and night, in the case of chronic illness, or more frequendy in acute conditions, care being taken that the bottle is previously **shaken 10 times** on each occasion. **8-10** doses, thus potentized, having been taken, a **fresh unused bottle** is provided and the remedy is administered again at a higher rate of dynamization, duly shaken 19 times before being taken.

In § 269 and 270, Hahnemann stresses the importance of dilution combined with dynamization by friction when trituration has been affected, and finally by succession. The number of shakes when the original remedy is prepared by a chemist should be 100, but for potions to be taken daily, 19 times on each occasion are prescribed, although the 5th edition stated that 2 sufficed. (See § 239, 247 footnote, § 240 and footnote, 270 and footnotes, 280 and 282).

There was a time when succussion was considered all-important. Then dilution was brought to play the lead-ing part. In the 6th edition Hahnemann ascribes the real efficacy of homoeopathic remedies to the combina-tion of these two' pharmacopractical factors, but he also lays stress on **the non-medicamental**

substratum, which enables the active substance to be dispersed and provides, as it were, by contact a new influence or energy (footnote to § 269).

3. **PHARMACONOMY**, or the channel of penetration of therapeutic agents, § 284 opens entirely new prospects as regards the channel of absorption of homoeopathic remedies:

i. **Oral absorption** through the mucous membrane of mouth, tongue, stomach and intestinal tube.

ii. **Inhalation** through the upper organs of respiration, nose and pharynx (and not olfaction as has quite erroneously been maintained) (§ 248, 284, 286)

iii. **Inspiration** through the lower organs of respiration, trachea, bronchi and lungs.

iv. **Friction** through the whole cutaneous surface of the body, **wherever the epidermis is sound** (a very important point) (§ 194 and § 284). It is a well known fact that any point of the epidermis covering is directly connected with the encephalic centres.

150 years ago, Hahnemann, much ahead of his times, suggested adopting as channels of absorption the oral and anal digestive tubes, a theory which is now considered the most modern. Whereas medicine absorbed through the mouth and swallowed may become partially inactive in the stomach or liver, the

perlingual absorption of medicine, as recommended by our master, may, by avoiding portal circulation, display its full efficacy upon the whole organism. The excellent innervation and the rich vascularization of the oral cavity, as well as the proximity of the large blood vessels and cervical sympathetic ganglia, provide perfect conditions for action through contact and good resorption with prompt effects. This was shown bv Hahnemann as early as 1810.

Inhalation through the upper and lower organs of respiration, which I have just described, has recently been practised in our modern "aerosols". Now, as regards friction through the cutaneous covering, it is known today that the parts of the epidermis through which the nervous centres may be reached may be divided into more or less privileged areas, corresponding to very definite parts of the encephalic centres. In the two earliest editions of the *Organon* Hahnemann had already alluded to the **epigastrium,** the **inner upper most of the thighs** and the **lower part of the abdomen as channels** for neuro-epidermic conduction to centres.

In § 284 and 285, he recommends non-systematic, but occasional friction, in the case of **very chronic complaints,** on back arms, thighs, and legs with the medicinal solution which has proved efficacious when administered internally. This, however, may only be resorted to **when the skin is perfectly sound** and free from **dermatoses, cramps or algies.** Whereas allopathy prescribes application of the drug to the affected parts, Homoeopathy advocates exactly the opposite.

Recent research is alleged to have shown that friction applied to the testicles or to the labia majora acts upon the pallido-cortical region. Some medicaments are even supposed to act more especially according to the part rubbed-(J Portie).

Hahnemann, as far as I know, never raised the question of **"time pharmaconomy"** (i.e. the most opportune moment of the 24 hours for the administration of a remedy) except in his **Materia Medica,** in his reference to **Nux Vomica.**

This question is also connected with the very delicate problem of **simultaneous intus et extra** application of a remedy. The local frictions recommended in § 284 and 285 would appear to be disapproved of in § 194, 196, 197, 198 and 199, where Hahnemann categorically rejects any application of or friction with any external remedy whatsoever on the diseased region in the course of an acute or chronic ailment localized by a dermatosis, a tumour, an area of vasoconstriction or vasodilatation. Any external application **loco-dolenti** is absolutely prohibited as being contrary to the doctrine. Hahnemann expounds his reasons in a very pertinent manner and, in the preface of his 6th edition, he states that only a perfectly healthy skin and treatment of a very chronic ailment can justify the simultaneous **intus et** extra application of a remedy.

4. I wish here to refer briefly to the important recommendation of Hahnemann, in § 265, to the effect that homoeopathic remedies should be **prepared and administered by the physician** or in his presence, in order to make sure that they are taken in the proper way. This is unfortunately a recommendation which modern physicians are hardly in a position to comply with.

5. We shall now approach the burning question of **HOMOEOPATHIC AGGRAVATION**

The careful observation which Hahnemann advocates after the administration of homoeopathic remedies is described in § 280 to 283 then further in § 155 to 161, 284, footnote to 253, 275 and 276. He deals therein with what we have called for the last 150 years **homoeopathic aggravation** and what modern classical medicine has recently detected and called **"rebound pheno-mena"**.

In his 6th edition, Hahnemann treats of **belated aggravation** (§161 and 248). This question is in close relationship with the two important ones dealt with in his last edition.

i. The appearance of **new symptoms** in the course of treatment and how to interpret them (§ 249 and 250).

ii. The limit of homoeopathic dynamization, dealt with in § 160, footnote to 249, and 279, and with regard to which Hahnemann asserts that there is **no limit to be set to the number of our dynamization as long as they can lead to aggravation.**

iii. On the subject of aggravation Hahnemann, who had already alluded without specifying (in § 138 and footnote to 210) to what is known as **the return of former symptoms,** comments upon this notion (which Kent was to deal with later in a magisterial way and gives an entirely modified version of it. This return, which J H Allen called **"retrograde metamorphosis"** is an extremely valuable indication for the homoeopath in making his prognosis.

The interpretation of new symptoms may be read with great interest as well as the therapeutic indications they provide, but, whether touch upon new symptoms or recurring ones, every thing reverts to **the reaction of the organism** on **the remedy,** with regard to which Hahnemann gives in his various paragraphs most enlightening data.

6. DYNAMIZATION

The important paragraph 270, though completely modified in the latest edition, asserts — as the *Organon* does whenever potencies are mentioned — that it is **centesimal** (§ 128, 270 and 271) and should always be effected in **separate phials,** which is indicated nowadays by the capital H following the figure relating to potency, 6H, 9H, 12H, 30H, etc, clearly showing that the preparation was done in separate bottles, unlike the system of the single bottle advocated by Korsakoff.

Hahnemann expounds:

i. New ideas on medicamental dispersion, associating **dilution** or simple dispersion of the substance, with **dynamization** or **potentialization** of latent medicinal properties by friction, trituration or succussion. **Homoeopathic remedies are not** inert substances whose **matter is divided** in the extreme. They are products which have been rendered essentially efficient by reinforcing their latent and highly disintegrated properties through a mechanical treatment which confers upon them new, active, and efficient properties (§ 269).

ii. Duration of the medicamental efficacy of homoeopathic remedies. In his last edition, Hahnemann asserts that these remedies may be kept for many years, provided they are sheltered from light and heat.

iii. Scales of concordances: As you all know, Hahnemann in the 5th edition, anticipating Mr Berne of Paris, had already attempted to shake a medicament for half an hour, believing thus to have multiplied by 30 the strength of the first centesimal dilution. When, however, he realized that he had been mistaken, he cancelled his former statement and replaced it by explanatory

notes in §270, where he describes the preparation of 50 millesimal, uniting the notions of quantity and quality.

iv. I have already mentioned above the problem of the limit of attenuation.

7. **PLACEBO**

In order to enable the physician to make a differential diagnosis distinguishing the worsening of the disease from that of the patient, Hahnemann, in § 96 and 281 (an innovation in the 6th edition), advocates recourse to **Placebo.**

8. **HOMOEOPATHY AND SOCIAL MEDICINE**

In the footnote to § 271 he outlines a social and philanthropic medical service whereby the sick, whether rich or poor, would be given free remedies through the bounty of the State.

9. **PRE- AND POST-NATAL HOMOEOPATHIC TREATMENT.**

The entirely new footnote, no 284 discusses:

i. The campaign against heredity by means of an antipsoric cure, the infant being treated **in utero** during pregnancy (the first, if possible), especially with **Sulphur.** "Thus it is much stronger and heal their at birth."

ii. The post-natal treatment called **"remedial nursing",** when the baby may be treated indirectly through its mother or foster-mother, who takes the remedy and transmits its properties to the baby through her milk.

"Just as a baby may contract psora through its foster-mother's milk, so it may be protected from it by the same milk once it has become a medicine owing to the antipsoric absorbed by the person giving suck."

10. Therapeutic creations after the first prescription, or differential diagnosis distinguishing symptoms recorded before treatment from those observed during it; enquiry into primal symptoms; importance of mental symptoms in the reaction; the imperative necessity for very minute dynamizations; all these are set out in the paragraphs revised nos. 91. 253, 255, 256.

11. Partial remedies and deficient diseases: Although § 162-170 for the former and 17 2-179 for the later have only been modified in some details, I would urge all homoeopaths carefully to read these articles on deficient diseases, since they are frequendy found among patients and are therapeutically of great significance.

Partial remedies are those whose pathogenesis has not been fully explored, but which apparently possess many therapeutic potentialities as yet unknown and undeveloped. Hahnemann shows us how to act in such cases, how to investigate symptomatic residues and reconsider cases after the first prescription.

Deficient diseases are those in which there is a dearth of symptoms. **The Organon** indicates what is to be done in such cases, of such daily occurrence in our consulting rooms.

Lack of symptoms should not be confused with want of practical knowledge on the part of the doctor, either because he does not give enough time to questioning his patient or because he is unable to detect the relevant symptoms. In that case it is not the disease which is deficient but the doctor.

12. Provings, or medicinal experimentation on a healthy man, now-a-days referred to as physiopathological investigation or, better still, human exploration.

How few doctors know that Hahnemann, in § 121-141, gave, with particular care and minuteness, all requisite details about the manner of experimenting with drugs on a healthy man! In that account you will find matter to satisfy the hunger and thirst of the seeker after knowledge: instructions for experimenting, dosage, diet, choice of the subject and his observation during proving, study of reactions, examination of the reports on the experiment, self-experimentation by the doctors, etc. Instead of trying, as in classical medicine, to interpret what goes on the laboratory (in vitro) which only comprises a limited number of parameters. Hahnemann has shown how to understand what is going on in vitro humano, where they are exceptionally numerous owing to the presence of a biologically suitable basis. There is no other means where-by one may thus "listen-in" to the human bios (what Hahnemann calls the dynamis) and infiltrate the field of human pathology in such a flexible and sensitive manner, for the bios is compounded of niceties and subtle inflexions. This matter of proving is one of the essential biological subterfuges of the human organism that lies concealed in it. Here, too, lies the fundamental link and hidden spring of Hahnemann's experimental method, for, by recommending the 30th potency as the starting-point for any proving, it enables the vital psychical symptoms of the subject to be disclosed at the outset.

The neuro-vegetative centres that compose the "ceiling" of the physiological entity form in exact coincidence the "floor" of the psychological entity, to which a modern allopathic writer, Portie, has given the name neuro-vegetative endo-consciousness.

These neuro-vegetative centres, which are to record all the valuable symptoms of the drug to be tested, are of great importance to us, for it is there that man's physiology and psychology meet: meet, and better still, coincide. Hahnemann's genious grasped the need to exploit the opening offered by this cardinal ambivalence which, from the neuro-vegetative centres to the endo-consciousness — coincident and identical, a Janus double — and yet single-visaged—operate the relays and transformations from the physiology to the psychology, that is, to the discursive intelligence which is thus infused, animated and adapted.

The experiment thus carried out is psychological as well as biological, hence the discursive exo-consciousness can become acquited with the incidents of the organic life.

Section 4: Defective Illnesesses

DEFECTIVE ILLNESSES

- Introduction
- Therapeutics of defective illness
- Reactive remedies of cardiopulmonary patients
- Reactive remedies for nervous subjects
- Reactive remedies of organic complaints
- Reactive remedies of cutaneous affections
- Reactive remedies of digestive states
- NOSODES

This is how I translate the expression 'Einseitige Krankheiten,' which we find interpreted in the other translations of the **Organon** into French, as "partial illnesses," which of course, is a mistake. This is what HAHNEMANN says in Paragraph 172: "A similar difficulty in the way of the cure occurs **from the symptoms of the disease being too few** - a circumstance that deserves our careful attention; for, by its removal, almost all the difficulties that can lie in the way of this most perfect of all possible modes of treatment (except that its apparatus of known homoeopathic medicines is still incomplete) are removed".

In Paragraph 162 HAHNEMANN had spoken of **fragmentary remedies** that have not been sufficiently tried which he calls: "Unvolkommene Arzneikrankheitspotenz".

In the next edition of the **Organon** it will be a good idea to complete the expression 'defective illnesses' and say, rather, 'natural defective illnesses', in contrast to these pathogenesis which have not been sufficiently developed.

Illnesses which show only one side, or one aspect, of their reality are called 'Einseitige Krankheiten'. We are not talking here about partial or fragmentary illnesses, because they are illnesses which involve and represent all of the individual; but we mean that they **do not show themselves completely**. That is why I have called them **defective illnesses**. On the other hand, "Unvolkommene Arzneikrankheits potenz" means 'incomplete pathogenetic dynamisation', which is a fragmentary drug that has not completely developed its action for want of sufficient proving, or for want of provers sensitive enough to react in all their faculties and organs: It isn't the fault of the drug, but of circumstances which have not allowed it to develop all its potential richness.

Paragraph 173: "The only diseases that seem to have but few symptoms, and on that account to be less amenable to cure, are those which may be termed **One-sided**, because they display only one or two principal symptoms, which obscure almost all the others. They belong chiefly to the class of chronic diseases."

Paragraph 174: "Their principal symptom may be either an internal complaint (e.g. a headache of many years duration, diarrhoea of long standing, an ancient cardialgia, etc.), or it may be an affection more of an **external kind**. Diseases of the latter character are generally distinguished by the name of **local maladies**."

The local illnesses, or the local maladies, which HAHNEMANN speaks about here, are in fact **localized illnesses**: The only local illnesses that we recognize in Homoeopathy are the result of traumatism. An eruption, a keratitis, an appendicitis, etc., are localized affections and not local. Among these localized maladies there are, for instance, warts, discolourations, intertrigo, strabismus, or squinting, aphthae, haemorrhoids, alopecia, etc.

We have therefore to consider three kinds of 'defective illnesses':

1. **Illnesses defective because of the patient**: Because there is a lack of real symptoms expressed by the patient. The patient tells you what is wrong with him: I can't sleep, I have no appetite, I feel tired. What can you do with symptoms like those? Nothing at all, because they are far too vague.

2. Illnesses defective because of the doctor: They are defective because of the lack of symptoms discovered and collected by the practicing homoeopath. In this case we must consider different insufficiencies:

a. **Insufficient questioning**: The doctor doesn't know the modalities and concomitants that he has to look for while questioning the patient.

b. **Ignorance of the four principles of questioning the patient:**

i. the doctor keeps interrupting his patient.

ii. the doctor asks direct questions to the patient which can only be answered by 'yes' or 'no'.

iii. the doctor asks questions grouped under two alternatives, obliging the patient to choose one of them.

iv. the doctor doesn't know really how to 'direct' the questioning!

c. Finally, there is the doctor who is too hurried. The patient has no time to answer because the doctor keeps asking questions too quickly; or else, if the patient is rather talkative, the doctor stops listening to him; or else he can't get an answer from a timid or an intimidated patient who does not dare to answer, or is too shy to answer. One must know how to encourage the patient to say everything that he wants to say. This is when we should repeat many times: Isn't there anything else? And what else? Haven't you forgotten anything? One must push the patient into a corner until he has nothing left to say at all. Only then can you start questioning him. Or, if it is taking too long, you can say to him: "That is very important. We will come back to that at a later date". After five or six consultations like that your patient will have exhausted everything he has to say.

But I insist that you take the trouble, before starting to question the patient, to ask him whether he is sure he has told you everything. If not, at the end of your consultation, you may see him pull a little paper out of his pocket and start reading it. Then the whole thing has to start again. If not, he may say to you (with what cheek): "Doctor, you have no time to listen to me, and I couldn't tell you everything!"

d. Then there is the doctor who interprets symptoms in his own way to simplify, or to save time, because he is in a hurry, leaving aside subjective symptoms and paying attention only to objective or immediately verifiable symptoms.

3. Finally, we have illnesses which are defective by their symptoms. These are illnesses which do not show themselves.

HAHNEMANN adds:

Paragraph 175: "In one-sided diseases of the first kind it is often to be attributed to the medical observer's want of discernment that he does not fully discover the symptoms actually present which would enable him to complete the sketch of the portrait of the disease."

Paragraph 176: "There are, however, still a few diseases, which, after the most careful initial examination (paragraphs 84-98), present but one or two severe, violent symptoms, while all the others are but indistinctly perceptible."

In this connection we must here remember the famous sixth paragraph of the **Organon** about the six categories you have to think about. Every homoeopath must know these six categories, which the doctor must constantly have in his mind.

Paragraph 6: "The unprejudiced observer - well aware of the futility of transcendental speculations which can receive no confirmation from experience - be his powers of penetration ever so great, takes note of nothing in every individual disease, except the changes in the health of the body and of the mind (**morbid phenomena, accidents, symptoms**) which can be perceived externally by means of the senses; that is to say, he notices only the deviations from the former healthy state of the now diseased individual, which are felt by the patient himself, remarked by those around him, and observed by the physician. All these perceptible signs represent the disease in its whole extent, that is, together they form the true and only conceivable portrait of the disease."

And then HAHNEMANN expounds these six categories:

1. First of all, there are those which come up during the questioning and are told by the patient himself. One must therefore listen to what he says (or read what he writes) about his personal feelings and let him takes as long as he likes. I insist on this. One must corner him completely until he has said everything he has to say.

2. Symptoms obtained and listed by questioning people around the patient. There are things that the patient doesn't say and which the doctor quite often doesn't see but that the people around the patient know; for instance, night convulsions or other manifestations that take place during sleep, little faults of character, signs in the gait, certain attitudes, etc.

3. Symptoms observed and noted by the doctor, with all the possible means at his disposal including x-rays, laboratory tests, physical examinations, and so on.

After his first symptom triad, HAHNEMANN gives us a second. Here again the first translation we have is wrong. The first translation of the **Organon**, in fact, tells us something which we have never understood, that is, that one recognizes illnesses in three manifestations: signs, accidents, and symptoms. I racked my brains for a long time trying to find out just what these three things meant. This, in fact, is what they mean.

4. Subjective symptoms felt by the patient himself, symptom often not objectively verifiable and very often minimized or neglected by the treating doctor. Homoeopathy is always interested in subjective symptoms because it is interested in the patient, in his personal reactions, in everything concerning him; while ordinary medicine is interested in objective symptoms, in the illness, to make a diagnosis, for which a treatment will subsequently be prescribed.

5. The signs are objective symptoms that can be measured, auscultated, felt, verified, identified, seen, and perceived, by all the means at our disposal either by our senses, or by the microscope, or all the apparatus used to detect symptoms or all the means known to the laboratory.

That is why, for us the homoeopaths; there are no illnesses without symptoms, because any illness which doesn't reveal itself to us through manifest symptoms can be discovered by laboratory techniques.

And the same thing applies, for accidents: The more blood there is, the more horrible it is and most of the time the less serious it is! But when we see just a small drop of blood coming from the ear or the nose, we know that it is much worse than something else which horrifies everybody around us. The small symptoms are always more important than the big ones. And in fact, it is the same in opthalmo-diagnosis. It isn't the big spots on the eye which are important but the very small details, sometimes hardly perceptible.

6. Accidents, unexpected symptoms, casual or accidental symptoms, all of them are symptoms occurring from accidents: burns, insect bites, wounds, etc.

We see, in addition, that 'defective illnesses' can present us with different possibilities:

1. There aren't enough symptoms, or not enough that can be considered usable.

2. There are too many symptoms. When you have a big muddle of symptoms, what can you do? I remember having questioned a patient when I was studying with Dr GLADWIN of Philadelphia. After questioning the patient for half an hour, which I thought was very thorough of me, and for which I even expected some congratulations. I had 40 symptoms, for which I had sweated..., in English! She rejected them, one after the other, not one of them being of any use... I was really

mortified. "You cannot", she said (for this was a female doctor, if you don't mind), "prescribe in any rational way on these symptoms because they are all common, too frequent, too vague, or too general: tiredness, depression, insomnia, headaches, constipation, and diarrhoea, without any modalities at all".

The patient may also make things up that didn't happen, and he gives you symptoms that you cannot make head or tail of, things that change each time. Still, we see very few patients who tell fibs or totally invent what they tell us!

3. There is also the question of symptoms that the patient won't tell you willingly because they are embarrassing, humiliating, shameful symptoms. You will find a remarkable description of these in the **Organon**, paragraph 93. It is up to the doctor to discover them with tact and psychology. I must tell you that opthalmo-diagnosis often helps us a great deal in this matter. I have often spoken about the flattening of the pupil at 12 o'clock: In the left eye it means sthenic manifestation, and in the right, asthenic, depressive. In the left eye it would indicate rage or repressed anger, for instance; in the right depression and sorrow.

I have already told you the story of the young woman who had one of the highest positions on the O.M.S. She was divorced because she had married a fellow quite beneath her, a sort of moron. After that she met a diplomat from Paris who courted her and promised to marry her. They were to marry at Christmas. She was very happy to have found, at last, someone worthy of her. And a few days before Christmas the suitor called her on the telephone and said that he unfortunately couldn't come, he had to leave, and wouldn't be there for the wedding! She never heard from him again.

She came to see me, saying, "Doctor, I am heartbroken!" I looked in her eyes. At the top, at 12 o' clock, in the right eye there was absolutely no flattening. In the left there was an enormous flattening. So I said to her: "You are not heartbroken at all. You feel enraged about your self-esteem, with repressed anger," Then she looked at me with tearful eyes and smiled, and said: "Yes, Doctor, I rather think you may be right!" And, of course, this was a case of *Staphysagria* not at all *Pulsatilla* or Ignatia.

So the examination of the eyes will allow you to discover mental symptoms that you cannot find in any other way.

We can also find very useful symptoms which the patients do not tell us without asking a single question, by observing the handwriting, the lines of the hand, the nails, the wrinkles of the face, the ears.

THERAPEUTICS OF DEFECTIVE ILLNESS

HAHNEMANN has the following to say about this:

Paragraph 177: "In order to meet most successfully such a case as **this**, which is of **very rare** occurrence, we are in the first place to select, guided by these few symptoms, the medicine which in our judgment is the most homoeopathically indicated".

A little before that he says in paragraph 166: "Such acase is, however, **very rare**, owing to the increased number of medicines whose pure effects are now known, and the bad effects resulting from it, when they do occur, are diminished whenever a subsequent medicine, of more accurate resemblance, can be selected".

This shows that most often it isn't only the patient's fault, but above all the doctor's fault. It is up to us to know our **Materia Medica** sufficiently well, to know what we have to ask.

I must say that the disciples of KENT have a great advantage. First, simply by opening KENT's **Repertory** they have a whole list of questions they can ask, which is to their advantage. Secondly, they know that all these questions have corresponding answers in the **Materia Medica**, which is another advantage. When we know our way around our repertory, we have there a considerable spectrum which allows us to ask questions that a doctor without a repertory cannot know, and therefore cannot ask, simply by relying on his memory. This is an enormous advantage over all other practitioners.

Paragraph 178: "It will, no doubt, sometimes happen that this medicine, selected in strict observance of the homoeopathic law, furnishes the similar artificial disease suited for the annihilation of the malady present. This is much more likely to happen when these few morbid symptoms are very striking, decided, uncommon, and peculiarly distinctive (characteristic)."

Paragraph 179: "More frequently, however, the medicine first chosen in such a case will be only partially, that is to say, not exactly suitable, as there was a small number of symptoms to guide to an accurate selection".

Now we come to the question of the so-called accessory symptoms, about which HAHNEMANN writes, as follows:

Paragraph 180: "In this case the medicine, which has been chosen as well as possible, but which, for the reason above stated, is only imperfectly homoeopathic, will, in its action upon the disease that is only partially analogous to it - just as in the case mentioned above (Paragraph 162, et. seq.), where the limited number of homoeopathic remedies renders the selection imperfect - produce accessory symptoms, and several phenomena from its own array of symptoms are mixed up with the patient's state of health, **which are, however, at the same time, symptoms of the disease itself, although they may have been hitherto never or very rarely**

perceived; some symptoms which the patient had never previously experienced appear, or others he had only felt indistinctly become more pronounced."

You see, HAHNEMANN thought of everything. These are revealing symptoms, which were hidden and now are laid bare. So you see that the expression 'partial illness' was not accurate.

These new symptoms can perhaps be linked to the secondary symptoms, or the iatrogenic symptoms of our allopathic colleagues, who are always striking the edge of toxicity with all their new drugs. After all, we must remember that allopathy is interested in finding out just how much of a drug the patient will tolerate:whereas we, the homoeopaths, deal in the minimum effective dose!

Paragraph 181: "Let us not object that the accessory phenomena and the new symptoms of this disease that now appear should be laid to the account of the medicament just employed. They owe their origin to it [1] certainly, but they are always only symptoms of such a nature as **this** disease was itself capable of producing in **this** organism, and which were summoned forth and induced to make their appearance by the medicine given, owing to its power to cause similar symptoms. In a word, we have to regard the whole collection of symptoms now perceptible as belonging to the disease itself, as the actual existing condition and to direct our further treatment accordingly".

Paragraph 182: “Thus the imperfect selection of the medicament, which was in this case almost inevitable owing to the too limited number of symptoms present,serves to complete the display of the symptoms of the disease, and in this way facilitates the discovery of a second, more accurately suitable, homoeopathic medicine”.

Paragraph 183: “Whenever, therefore, the dose of the first medicine ceases to have a beneficial effect (if the newly developed symptoms do not, by reason of their gravity, demand more speedy aid - which, however, from the minuteness of the dose of homoeopathic medicine, and in very chronic diseases, is excessively rare), a new examination of the disease must be instituted, the status morbi as it now is must be noted down, and a second homoeopathic remedy selected in accordance with it, which shall exactly suit the present state, and one which shall be all the more appropriate can then be found, as the group of symptoms has become larger andmore complete. [2]

This is something which KENT often repeats. You have given a remedy and the result isn’t brilliant. Instead of starting immediately to give a whole lot of other drugs, question your patient again, complete your examination and you will see that quite often the remedy will manifest itself without any difficulty.

In addition, this paragraph raises the question of lack of reaction; if we have proceeded as we should ...

Here it is well to remember that we must differentiate between two categories of reactions:

The drug has been really well chosen, based on a serious case-taking. Its origin and preparation leave no doubt about its effectiveness; it corresponds to the patient's real symptoms of the moment. In this case HAHNEMANN indicates *Opium*, if there is a lack of reactions. You know that *Opium* paralyzes, stops all reactions, whether nervous, muscular, or sphincteroid. That is why, according to Dr. FLURY, when a doctor is called to a case of hepatic or renal colic at night and makes an injection of morphine, he always goes home disgusted, annoyed, and dissatisfied with himself; but, if he has been able to find the right remedy and relieve the patient - and this is perfectly possible - then it is quite a different story and he has a clear conscience.

In KENT's **Repertory** on page 1397 there is the rubric; 'Lack of Reaction", you will look back to page 1369: "Lack of Irritability', and you will add to the rubric on page 1397: *Bryonia, Calc-iod.,* Cypripedium, **Tub**., X-ray, **Zinc**.

And when too many drugs have produced a state of hypersensitivity and the remedy fails, you have to think of *Ph-ac*., and above all ***Teucr.*** (page 1369).

On page 1288, in intermittent fever that has been spoiled by a whole lot of drugs, you have a rubric which indicates several drugs, among which you find *Sepia*, and you find it listed equally on page 1282.

Now we come to a whole series of precisions, very useful in practice, which allow us to choose the **reactive** remedy properly. These reactive remedies will either open up the case, bring about an initial improvement that can be followed up later on, or else, more often, they will not seem to produce any immediate result; but afterwards the patient will feel an indefinable improvement in himself, and a repetition of the drug, which started the improvement in the beginning, and then seemed to stop acting will bring about a new improvement and sustain that improvement. Thus the flame will be rekindled, and the favorable reaction, which was interrupted, will be revived and strengthened once again.

Therefore we shouldn't believe, or expect, that the reactive remedy will bring about an immediate result. Sometimes there will not be any apparent result, but the real remedy of the patient will once again be able to act. A general rule is not to repeat the reactive remedy. We give it only once and see what happens, or, as the English say: Watch and wait.

After the reactive remedy how long should one wait? Usually three to five days, or even longer, if there is a good result (and in that case continue as usual allowing the improvement to run its course). But, if you have no result, wait three to five days without repeating the original drug.

REACTIVE REMEDIES OF THE AGED

In KENT's **Repertory** look under 'Old People' or 'Aged People' or 'Old Age'.

An elderly person is someone who is at least over 65, although certain patients are old long before that, and, on the other hand, others who have reached 75, are still very young. Therefore this is a question of discrimination which you will have to make for yourself.

There are two excellent reactive remedies for elderly persons: *Ambra grisea* and *Teucrium marum verum*, which you will give if you have some symptoms indicating them, and I shall speak about that now.

Ambra grisea: Is suitable especially for elderly people and patients who are weakened by age, or as a result of over-work.

These people are hypersensitive, exhausted, nearly always have insomnia because of worry, and have to get up at night.

Usually there is aggravation from music, which they do not like and which makes them weep.

Crotchety and fussy, they hate anything which is out of the ordinary routine of their lives and disturbs their habits. Like *Cann-i.* and *Glon.*, for them time passes too slowly (if it passes too quickly, *Cocc.*). They are nervous, intensely shy, and cannot do anything in the presence of someone else. They desire to be alone.

Nervous and excitable infants; loquacious subjects; a great remedy for elderly people disgusted with life; people hating strangers and everything new.

These patients usually suffer on one side only, usually the **right side**, but also the right side on top and the left side at the bottom. When certain subjects have symptoms only on one side, and you cannot find those symptoms listed on page 1400 of the **Repertory**, under the right or the left side, whichever the case may be, then you should look at the first rubric, **'Symptoms on One Side only**', without worrying about whether it is the right or the left side.

Ambra symptoms further include:

Vertigo of the aged and loss of hair.

Epistaxis, aggravated in the morning; much bleeding of the gums.

Frequent feeling of coldness on the abdomen.

Spasmodic cough with eructation; aggravated in the presence of others;

A loose, deep hacking cough with palpitations;

Nymphomania;

Pruritis of the sexual organs;

Tendency to metrorrhagia;

Cramps in the hands and in the fingers.

Teucrium marum verum:When the great number of drugs administered has produced a state of hypersensitivity, with the result that no remedy, even if it is indicated, acts. Specific action on the nose and the rectum. Generally speaking patients who need *Teucrium* usually have:

Dry, chapped skin and have suffered in their infancy (or still suffer) from mucouspolyps somewhere in the nose or the nasopharynx, or the womb, or the bladder, or the rectum.

Childhood complaints.

A nose that is always stuffy.

Ozæna.

Anosmia.

Coryza with blocked nose.

One of the remedies that have the sensation of 'internal trembling'

These patients are prone to hiccups and nearly always have the post-nasal passage blocked.

Constant hiccough while eating or after lactation.

Musty taste in the mouth.

REACTIVE REMEDIES OF CARDIOPULMONARY PATIENTS

In this section there are five remedies which are especially important.

First of all: *Carbo vegetabilis*:

This remedy is a classic for subjects who have never recovered their health after a serious illness (pneumonia, typhoid, grippe, etc.). This is one of those cleansing remedies, a great 'drainer'! In that case give 10M potency, which works particularly well. A reactive remedy for defective reactions. It is also indicated after strong allopathic 'drugging'.

Remember that in the *Carbo veg.* patient everything is cold: the end of the nose; the extremities, hands and feet, face, teeth, mouth, breath, integuments - not only cold, even icy, except for the head, which is often hot. In spite of this typical cold, with venostasis, cyanosis, these patients quite paradoxically often have:

Feelings of local and regional burning.

Carbo veg. is anxious, especially in the evenings, in bed, on closing the eyes. He presents three very different, but very characteristic states: discouragement; indifference to everything, without reaction; irritability.

Generally speaking, collapse and all kinds of fainting following the loss of vital fluids.

Stagnation of blood in the capillaries, causing simple ecchymosis, cyanosis, haemorrhage of all the mucous membranes.

Septicaemia.

Asthenia, exhaustion, debility; easy fainting, for instance, in the morning upon getting up.

Aggravated by **fatty food, butter, pork, rich food**.

Heavy head, as if squeezed; hat feels too heavy.

Hot head, breath cold.

Hair falls out easily.

Black "muscae volante" before the eyes.

Dry ears or ears with too much wax.

Epistaxis every day; **black blood.**

Cyanosis of the face; chlorotic; pale, pasty; unhealthy look.

Hippocratic facies.

Cold sweat of the face, mottled cheeks, and the tip of the nose red.

Cracked lips; gums that bleed easily, especially when they are sucked.

Amelioration from eructation of wind, especially after **butter** and acids.

Stomach cramps which fold the patient in half, half an hour after eating, aggravated in summer.

Stomach burning and morning nausea.

Desire for **salty things**.

Aggravation from all fatty food.

Frequent indigestion; very sensitive epigastrium.

Painful diarrhoea of elderly people.

Glutinous secretions at the anus which burn, aggravated by scratching.

Green leucorrhea; early menses; prolonged menses.

Excellent remedy at the beginning of whooping cough.

Wheezing respiration.

Carbo veg. nearly always feels weight on the chest; constantly oppressed; frequent need to fan himself; needs the windows wide open; he needs air so badly that he asks for something with which to fan himself.

Sighing and irregular breathing.

Faint, feeble, imperceptible pulse.

Hoarse voice, no pain, aggravated in the evening.

Weak voice, especially singing high notes, aphonia.

Coryza with cough.

Cold hands, knees, legs, worse at night.

Prunus laurocerasus:For cardiovascular complaints with cyanosis and dyspnoea. **Cyanosis and rales in the newborn.**

The cold is not ameliorated by heat; he always has his hand on his heart.

This is the typical **snorer**, with very deep sleep (catapnoea). As far as the snoring is concerned, and the stertorous respiration, this remedy rivals *Opium* and *Lac caninum*, which are the two remedies which have the most snoring (or the best).

This reminds me of a story of my dear mother, who was still very active at 82 when she returned here in March from a trip to Cannes. Eight days later I went to see her one morning and rang her doorbell. No reply. Fortunately, I had a key. I went in, saw the kitchen, the sitting room, empty. No mother! Where could she be? That was when I heard a dreadful snoring. I went into her room and found her in bed, eyes closed, absolutely passed out, with the rale of the dying. Alas, I know that rale very well.

Speaking of this, I must tell you that this is something that always worries people around the sick. I saw that in my Master, who was dying when I was in

India. Many nervous and agitated adepts were around me and begged me to do something to calm him down, give him a shot of morphine - which he would never have allowed. I simply turned his head a little to one side, and the rale immediately stopped. Therefore it was enough simply to modify a little the position of the head! For people who snore when they sleep at night it is quite a different story. Often they have an elongation of the uvula, and when they lie down, especially if they lie very low, the uvula vibrates in the back of the throat. This disturbs many people, especially the wife, who is furious because she can't sleep; whereas her husband sleeps with his fists closed, snoring! There are special little structures which one can fix on the neck and the head, and which hold the chin and do not allow it to drop; but husbands do not readily accept this imposition, as you can imagine.

Yet, I once knew a great lawyer at the International Court at the Hague, a director and president of many commissions and congresses; but he was like a little boy before his wife. She made him wear this sort of mask, which stopped his chin from falling when he slept. The poor man hated it but he had to take it!

This method is usually not very popular. Snorers can use an extra cushion behind their backs so that the whole thorax is higher and the airway functions without obstruction. One can also wear a belt with a big knot in the back which will force one to sleep on one's side, and this lessens the condition.

Well, I found my poor mother in this state. I lifted the blankets and looked for reflexes; there were none in any part of the body. I lifted her arm, it fell back heavily. I took a pin and tested her sensitivity by pricking her more or less deeply, evoking no movement at all. The pupils were very small and hardly reacted to light. What was I to do? I thought that at 80 one had the right to die in peace; so I called a nurse to look after her; and there was nothing for the nurse to do.

Three days later my 19 year old niece, who studies biology and works in a laboratory, said to me: "Really, you homoeopaths make me sick! Half of your remedies are only make-believe! That is why you leave your patients to die with their arms crossed on their chests. Do something, an injection of strychnine or camphor or anything at all, but do something!" We had a dreadful argument, but I thought that perhaps there was something in Homoeopathy that one could give. When you see someone who doesn't move and has no reflexes, with a very small pupil, and who snores, and is completely unconscious, what picture does that bring to mind? Well, you must be an infant in arms not to think of *Opium*.

So I gave my mother a 200th potency of *Opium*, just a few tiny globules on the tongue. Ten minutes later I saw her left eye open and close and her right eye do the same thing. Half an hour later her eyelids started fluttering, then movements appeared in the upper limbs. The first night she urinated, and the intestines rendered unto Caesar that which was Caesar's. In a word, in the evening she had reflexes and her pupils had become larger. I gave her three doses in all and the result was extraordinary and spectacular. Eight days later she was sitting up, spoke a little, although with difficulty. And a month later, would you believe it, she was gathering flowers on the Petit Salève Mountain! She lived three years after that. I wonder what our dear colleagues would have done? No doubt, injections of Camphor, or Coramine, or God knows what else; and certainly they wouldn't have any result except to send her off from Charybdis to Scylla.

Hydrocyanic acid: A great cardiovascular drug, which is often forgotten; and yet it has always given me remarkable results. It is one of the most toxic and most mortal poisons!

For the mental symptoms, it is an interesting drug. It is a great frightener, fear of everything.

It also has cyanosis, with collapse, but more pulmonary than cardiac; while *Carbo veg.* and *Laurocerasus* have more effect on the heart.

Suffocation and constriction of the chest.

Palpitations.

Angina pectoris

The pulse is slow and flabby.

Sensation of emptiness, epigastric region.

Foaming at the mouth.

You always have to look at the pupil; the pupil of *Hydrocyanic acid* is dilated and without reaction.

Ammonium carbonicum: These patients don't like cleanliness at all. You may be sure that they use neither brush nor soap. They hate water and hate using it. This doesn't mean that you will give this remedy only to patients who are dirty.

This remedy presents an absolute incompatibility with *Lachesis*, and you have to know this incompatibility. You can have serious accidents if you give *Lachesis* after *Ammonium carb.*, in the hope of getting a reaction... just try it!

This patient is usually sedentary.

Big people, always tired, exhausted for no reason at all, with heaviness of all the organs.

Hates cold air.

Doesn't even like to touch water, let alone cold water! *Sulphur* doesn't like to be washed.

Ammonium carb. doesn't like it either but he actually fears the contact with water, which he hates.

Always has to carry a bottle of smelling salts to avoid fainting, or swooning!

Epistaxis after washing the face or the hands, and after eating; especially at night.

Marked tendency to catch cold.

Nose always blocked. The nose is especially blocked at night.

Lips cracked; cracks in the corners of the mouth; a crack in the middle of the lower lip.

Wakes up every morning sneezing. I have a patient who said: "My husband is unbelievable! I always know what time it is because at exactly seven o'clock in the morning suddenly I hear him sneeze. He wakes me up!" One dose of *Ammonium carb.* (and you will find that it is in the third degree in the **Repertory**) succeeds in most instances.

Creaking of the jawbone in chewing.

Bleeding haemorrhoids, aggravated during menses.

Anal pruritis.

Protruding haemorrhoids during stool.

Very frequent menses, profuse, with great tiredness.

Pungent, abundant, burning leucorrhoea, milky and smelling of ammonia.

Aversion to the opposite sex.

Involuntary urination at night.

A feeling of fullness in the head.

Patients who are rather obese, with a large appetite.

Audible palpitations; they say that they can hear their heart beating! Angina pectoris.

This subject is rather chesty, asthmatic, always out of breath, with noisy breathing that is more or less audible.

Great remedy of emphysema. The oppression is noticed particularly in climbing, but also on entering a hot room.

All chest symptoms are always aggravated at three o'clock in the morning.

All the pains are ameliorated by external pressure.

Whitlow.

Heaviness of all the internal organs.

It is a remedy for uraemia, don't forget this. It antidotes adrenalin.

Tarentula hispanica: This drug is very much neglected, and it is a pity: First of all, it is one of the most agitated of the drugs. He can't sit still, he can't stay in one place, must move about, especially at night.

Syndrome of the legs that will not rest, constantly fidgeting. You must remember also that this fidgeting is both physical and mental.

The agitation is often anxious.

Aversion to company, but patients who respond to *Tarentula* always want someone near to them, ready to help them.

Always dissatisfied.

Capricious.

Very changeable moods. These people are difficult to live with, whether children or adults.

Precordial anguish with constriction.

Palpitations with the feeling that the heart is being squeezed.

Immediate amelioration from music! That is why in my consulting rooms I have a button I can press to switch on a recording of music. When I have restless children, who run all over the room, I press the button, and as if by a miracle they stop, calm down, and listen! This is a very good indication for *Tarentula*.

Yearly periodicity.

REACTIVE REMEDIES FOR NERVOUS SUBJECTS

Gelsemium sempervirens: You know that in English you can sum up this remedy with three 'D's':

Dizzy,

Drowsy,

Dull.

When you see somebody, especially after flu, who is dizzy, and always drowsy, no thirst, apathetic, dull, think of this remedy.

Gelsemium has always light-colored urine, never dark, even when there is fever. And if you prescribe *Gelsemium* for a patient who has dark urine, that will prove that you are extremely defective and have a great need to take a refresher course!

Frequent urination, abundant urination which relieves headache.

A great remedy for trembling, but I draw your attention to this:external trembling. One can say that many *Gelsemium* patients, especially feverish patients, complain that everything is trembling.

The pulse is abnormal, slow but full, intermittent, irregular. It can also be rapid and tachycardia, feeble, soft, almost imperceptible, aggravated by movement. It is these apparent contradictions that make the charm and the value of our **Materia Medica**.

You know that this is the remedy for bad news, and you remember the story [3] of the patient I spoke about before who was overtaken with a dreadful buzzing of the ears when he received a bad news, the sudden death of one of his friends, whom he had recently seen.

And he was brilliantly cured with this remedy, while our allopathic colleagues had energetically treated him without the slightest little result... quite the contrary! Every time a patient tells you that he has had a sudden sorrow, ask him how it started. Often it comes from the shock of some bad news. In such cases always prescribe a high potency: *Gelsemium* 10M. If, on the other hand, this is a case of real sorrow, rather give *Ignatia*; and speaking of that, I have had cases which came back and reproached me afterwards: "Doctor, it is quite dreadful, you gave me a homoeopathic remedy so that I would be sustained under the emotion of a great bereavement; I went to the funeral and, although I am so sensitive, I couldn't even cry!"

Aggravated by all emotions. A great fearful remedy. Always a terrible fear before examinations. This is very successful when it is prescribed as a specific for fear of examinations. I give a dose of the 200th the morning of the examination, and if this fear of the examination is very pronounced, a dose even the day before in the evening. More often than not that is admirably successful; I don't even have to repeat it afterwards. What an advantage and what a blessing, especially in pipe organ examinations, when one's foot trembles on the great bass pedals... to make even the examiner tremble;and as for singing... when you **can't get a sound out**, *Gelsemium* maintains the voice of a nightingale!

So *Gelsemium* is very apprehensive.

Very frightened especially frightened of death. Remarkable after fear and emotions.

Wants to be left in peace.

Agoraphobia, fear of walking across large open spaces.

Fear of being alone, wants someone near, even someone who doesn't speak.

Fear of going in mountain cableways and elevators, even going down!Terrified of everything unexpected. Fear of falling.

Fear of losing his self-control and his calmness.

Fear of lightning; what a dreadful coward!

A real living barometer. *Gelsemium* very quickly feels all the fluctuations of the weather, especially when the barometer falls.

Constantly aggravated by thinking of his troubles.

But be careful, he unfortunately always feels better when he has had alcohol to drink!I had a patient once, who had this unfortunate peculiarity with, in addition, all the other symptoms of *Gelsemium*. She used to say to me: "Doctor, you wouldn't believe it, a friend of mine told me about this: I take the tiniest possible glass of 'kirsch' every morning, and afterwards it is absolutely marvellous, I feel that I have wings all day long to do the house work". That is really dangerous. She started with a tiny little glass, and a year later it was a litre of '**kirsch**' that she drank every morning. Her liver, especially, suffered from this, as you can well imagine. She developed dropsy with a whole lot of complications and she died of anasarca in the greatest moral and material misery! The constant repetition of her vice immediately antidoted the action of *Gelsemium!*

Fear of death. Feeble, slow pulse, even imperceptible.

Capsicum annuum: This drug is not chilly, as you will see it stated in many **Materia Medicas**, but on the other hand is **aggravated by the cold** and the slightest draft, which is an important nuance you have to remember.

Capsicum patients are flabby, **obese, lazy**; they want to be left in peace; these patients are apathetic and are always down. I promise you that you will never find them breaking speed limits. **Lack of reaction in obese patients**.

These people love routine and they hate anything unexpected. Write it in your repertory under the heading '**Unexpected, Aversion to Anything**'. If you tell them that you will take them on a drive tomorrow, they won't like that at all. You will have to tell them long in advance.

Great difficulty getting going to go out or to go on a drive or a walk. They hate all exercise and all effort.

And yet, **amelioration once they start to walk.**

Capsicum is an overworked intellectual who doesn't eat enough and is always in need of stimulants and tonics. **Dyspepsia of elderly people**.

It is a funny thing that this patient is always **thirsty after stool!!** And his scrotum is cold in the morning on waking up!

Like *Ammonium carbonicum* this remedy isn't very fond of cleanliness; you will see that their clothes are dirty, their ties have spots on them, and they are always improperly washed or shaven! Ugh!

Constantly dissatisfied and complaining.

This drug is indicated for a special illness, for which Allopathy is absolutely useless unless you go through two years of psycho-analysis... It is homesickness. This drug is especially recommended for young maidservants who have bright cheeks and who suddenly tell you after two weeks of their new job that they cannot stay and want to go home... A little dose of *Capsicum* 10M on the tongue of the young girl will bring back a smile and the pleasure of serving you! The Germans make fun of these symptoms and say: "These homoeopaths are quacks... they prescribe *Capsicum* for red cheeks and homesickness... It seems quite ridiculous..." But since it works I am very happy to use this remedy when it is indicated in this way, and I would very much like to know what an orthodox physician would do in such a case. You can't get anywhere, and the young maidservant goes home. Everything is overthrown for her and for everybody else! So this is a great remedy in cases of homesickness.

Hates drafts.

Explosive cough, as if everything were going to explode: head, ears, bladder, and chest. Sciatica aggravated from coughing. **Hoarse, raucous voice of public speakers, ministers, and singers.**

There is a localization for which this remedy is very successful: the mastoid. One or two doses of the 200th potency and the threatening mastoiditis disappear rapidly. This remedy acts very quickly and very well. Smokers and drinkers who suffer from sore throat and pains that goes to the ears, with fetid breath.

Valeriana officinalis: When it is dynamised, this plant has an affinity with subjects who have an extremely variable temperament. The height of instability. I don't mean alternating moods; I mean variable and irritable moods.

Impressionable, hypersensitive, very nervous.

Asthenic. **Hysterical complaints.**

Pulse generally accelerated.

Nervous system always rather excited.

This remedy has the sensation as if there were a thread hanging in the throat!

Excellent drug for babies who vomit great pieces of curdled milk after feeding.

Calcarea ostrearum: We must not use *Calcarea carbonica* which is indicated in all the books and is a chemical carbonate of lime, but, if we are serious homoeopaths, the living calcium, which is called *Calcarea ostrearum,* and is made by the oyster in the middle layer of his shell. If we want to go one step further in subtlety, we always use only those remedies which have been prepared from sources which were used for the provings.

But Providence is so generous that even if we practice Homoeopathy 'badly', even if we haven't got 'perfect' remedies we can still achieve extraordinary results. Really, our needs have been abundantly filled, and we should be grateful.

Calcarea ostrearum is the great homoeopsoric of HAHNEMANN. It covers all three miasms, and *Calcarea* is a remedy which we cannot do without. It is a part of the cycle *Sulphur-Calcarea-Lycopodium*, and therefore should never be given after *Lycopodium* nor before *Sulphur*. That would mix up the case to such a degree that it would be very difficult later on to clear it up. KENT said that there were certain patients who could never be restored because this rule had not been observed in their case. In the same way one should never go directly from *Sulphur* to *Lycopodium* one must find an intermediary drug to give between the two. These little points of advice of old, seasoned homoeopaths must really be respected!

The leucophlegmatic type, who, to speak from a hormonal point of view, has a thyroid-pituitary dysfunction.

Produces goitres... and cures them!

Great remedy for very shy people.

Has many fears, like *Phosphorous*. And my teachers taught me that when any case has more than three fears, one can almost always say that either *Calcarea* or *Phosphorous* is indicated. On condition, of course that we are not speaking about a mental case because it is very difficult in those cases to eliminate everything which can be pathognomonic?

He is very much afraid of: illness and contagion, epidemics, falling ill, suffering, tuberculosis, heart disease, being observed.

He is afraid of spirits, of losing his reason, disaster, losing his position, he is sure that a disaster will happen.

He is afraid of: poverty, dying of hunger, obscurity, night, evenings, and above all, twilight.

He is afraid of: being in bed, dogs, being in a crowd, animals, being alone, lightning and above all, death.

He is horrified on hearing stories of cruelty.

I have already told you the story of Dr. MATTOLI who was a man just as small as he was intelligent, a brilliant mind who spoke with great facility, and what volubility! - all this, of course, in magnificent Italian. One would have thought it was DANTE speaking: and when he was speaking, even if you didn't understand Italian, it was a pleasure to listen to him. Well, Dr. MATTOLI was once president of a congress in Rome when Mussolini was in power. The first day we were all assembled in an extraordinary hall with flags of different colours, old paintings, sculptures, beautiful armchairs, and we heard the President of the Ligue, Dr. GAGLIARDI, presenting to us a case of mental illness which had been cured by *Calcarea*. His description was perfect: he made of this expose something so marvellous from a scientific and literary point of view, that from the sixth row, where there were some allopaths who had been invited to the congress, one suddenly heard someone exclaim, 'Miracolo'! That's how marvellous his description was! Then, suddenly like a devil jumping out of a basin of holy water, Dr MATTOLI got up and said: "Who says it was a miracle?" Then these colleagues of ours got up and nodded - I mean the allopaths we had invited! MATTOLI continued: "Well, gentlemen, I must say, you are the only ones who make miracles, not us". And these gentlemen were very pleased, even more puffed up with pride, delighted with this compliment! MATTOLI continued: "Because, what is a miracle? A miracle is something exceptionally rare, which doesn't happen often. But for us homoeopaths, successes like this happen every day! And that is why we don't call them miracles!!"Sustained applause throughout the hall!You can imagine the effect of this interruption!

Calcarea is full of many fears; there are 26 different ones in KENT's Repertory! In addition, *Calcarea* is very forgetful. He also despairs of recovery (like some other drugs). **Anxiety at dusk**.

Very much indicated in convalescence that is not getting on and for patients who continually relapse.

Very wilful infants with a tendency to obesity.

There is a special sweating which is always regional, localized! - especially in the front of the body; and he perspires at night. He also sweats when he is anxious or after eating, or at the slightest exertion, or even from mental activity.

Look at the pupils. *Calcarea* is often mydriastic like *Belladona*, its acute. **Eyelids glued together in the morning**.

Tumultuous palpitations at night; after eating; with the slightest exertion, especially on climbing the stairs; also during fever.

Aversion to movement and exercise—a very lazy schoolboy who will ask to be let off gym practice!

He can't stand fasting or skipping a meal. And yet, he always feels worse after eating! Isn't it hard to reconcile these paradoxes! **Diarrhoea and vomiting at teething**.

Desire for eggs, and particularly hard-boiled eggs.

As a child he prefers and enjoys things that are rather strange and indigestible: chalk, carbon, pencil leads, etc. He loves sour fruit and, above all, ice cream.

He hates fat and two more things: coffee and meat. That doesn't mean that you must never give *Calcarea* to someone who likes coffee. There are other symptoms which will indicate it, and you can't possibly expect to find all the symptoms that *Calcarea* will cause and cure!

You know that classic symptom of *Calcarea* - horrible visions at the moment of falling asleep. He sees scowling faces! This symptom is very useful for prescription.

Amelioration from constipation, which is a rare symptom but a precious one, and unless I am mistaken, a symptom which is to be found in only two other remedies besides *Calcarea*. Look for them in the Repertory and don't forget them!

Calcarea infants sometimes have enormous stool, and one wonders how it is possible for infants to expel such stools!

When a patient who smokes suddenly loses his taste for cigars or cigarettes, think of *Calcarea*.

This remedy loves good wine, liqueurs, cold drinks, but on the other hand prefers milk when it is very hot! He loves everything which is salty or sour. It is a very good remedy if, in addition to these general characteristics, the patient suffers from polyps or exostoses.

REACTIVE REMEDIES OF ORGANIC COMPLAINTS

For the sequelae of paralysis, apoplexy, exhaustion, all cerebrospinal affection, depressions, asthenia, there are three remedies we have to think of above all; *Zincum, Conium,* and *Helleborus.*

Zincum metallicum: One word sums it up: **exhausted** (overworked, broken down). As the English put it, 'fag'. This patient has no more vitality: he is completely prostrated, can't go on: he is exhausted: he has capitulated!

As soon as he becomes ill he is immediately depressed, immediately thinks of the worst. *Zincum* straight-away thinks of everything in the blackest terms! **Spinal affections.**

There is an etiological symptom that you must know because it always succeeds very well and is very precious for us homoeopaths, who usually have to treat the leftovers of Allopathy. We nearly always see cases which have been treated, manhandled, spoiled, complicated... and when we cure them we are told that this is imagination! When you have **an eruption which has been suppressed, a discharge which has been stopped by nitrate of silver, by suppositories, or by ointment, etc.** *Zincum* is the king of all such situations. In those cases we see the discharge reappearing, the eruption flowering anew, and the patient feeling better.

In a case of measles, scarlet fever, any eruptive fever, any **eruptive illness which doesn't end properly**, give a dose of *Zincum* and immediately you see the eruption coming back. Remember that *Zincum* **ameliorates every discharge** wherever it is: excretions, urine, diarrhoea, suppurations, menses, etc...

Every patient with trembling, tics, myoclonus, spasms. Syndrome of legs that cannot stop fidgeting. Agitation when seated; pupils who constantly move their legs during class!

Hypersensitive to noise and above all the sound of voices, which put him beyond himself! The child repeats questions that are put to him and everything one says to him.

Like *Sulphur*, he has a **sudden ravenous hunger at 11 o'clock in the morning**. If he goes home at about 11 o'clock he immediately looks for something to eat because he can't wait for lunch...

Zincum **cannot stand wine**. **Cephalalgia from alcohol**.

The **pulse is rapid**, especially in the evening, and it is **intermittent**. This is an objective symptom which can be useful in defective illnesses.

Very good action on pterygia; itching of the internal canthus, which is often irritated; rolls his eyes; looks cross-eyed.

Pale complexion; angular cheilitis at the corners of the mouth; tendency to hawk.

Children who constantly move their legs for fear of urinating, who lose their urine while walking or coughing or sneezing.

The loss of pubic hair in both sexes.

Pains of the left ovary; sensitive breasts, especially during menses; menses more abundant at night; complaints that are noticeably ameliorated during the menses.

For those whose legs fidget during sleep;

Itching of the thighs and especially of the popliteal spaces.

It is a great remedy for varicose veins of the lower extremities which are aggravated during pregnancy; chilblains of the extremities; somnambulism.

All the results of eruptions having been suppressed by ointments, lotions, radiations, all other external means.

Conium maculatum: This is an old remedy which has become a classic, thanks to PLATO, because it was used to put SOCRATES to death.

It is the **remedy of bachelors** and of old maidservants... the type that likes to be alone and hates visitors. He hates people he doesn't know because he is shy.

Hypochondriac, indifferent, not interested in anything; **averse to all intellectual work** and also to **all physical effort**. Weakness, decline, **laziness**. It is very difficult for him to come to the point of starting to do anything. He **cannot walk quickly**; he cannot hurry; and if you want to go with him you will have to proceed at his pace, which is always slow.

He always **feels better when he can let his arms or his legs hang!** Here we have another one of those things that may seem useless and unimportant, and yet for an informed homoeopath it will allow him to select the right remedy!

Heavy, stiff legs; difficult walking.

Neoplastic and arteriosclerotic diatheses.

The **head spins**, often with headache, and always **aggravated from lying down.** A great characteristic of the dizziness of *Conium* is the **amelioration from closing the eyes**.

Pronounced photophobia to all light, but without inflammation of the conjunctiva. Aversion to light without any affection of the eyes.

The cough is aggravated on lying down; and when he starts to cough at night in his bed, *Conium* **must sit up**. Coughing from irritation from a little dry point in the larynx, aggravated lying down; must sit up.

The pulse of *Conium* is accelerated after stool; it can also be small, intermittent, and irregular.

Interrupted urination. The urinary stream stops, then starts again!

Palpitation after every defecation.

The results of sexual repression in both sexes.

Sexual desire without erection.

Swelling of the breasts, with bruising pains, from touch, especially in front, but also during menses.

Perspiration as soon as he falls asleep, and even as soon as he closes his eyes. Excess of wax in the ears.

These patients feel better with the arms and the legs hanging.

Helleborus niger: This drug brings about sensorial depression with a bitter insipid taste. Fetor oris. Movements of chewing; food always tastes insipid, or else bitter. In all illnesses, absence of thirst.

Encephalic cry, especially at night while sleeping.

Convulsions of nursing infants.

Melancholic subjects who are always slow to answer when spoken to. Involuntary sighing. Dull, apathetic, indifferent.

Loss of hair and of the nails.

Mydriasis. Fixed stare without any reason.

Cold sweat on the face.

Always rubbing his nose.

These patients always have diminished vitality. And they have two things that you will notice: anasarca and dropsy. Like *Belladonna* and *Tuberculinum*, *Helleborus* always **bores the head into the pillow**. And he **rolls his head on the pillow** day and night. They eyeballs always gaze upward. Hemeralopia.

Carphological movements during pain.

A very good remedy for patients who get **goose flesh**.

Frequent and ineffective urging to urinate.

The pulse is generally rapid, faint, and trembling, it can also sometimes be slow.

REACTIVE REMEDIES OF CUTANEOUS AFFECTIONS

Zincum metallicum: The remedy of choice for the results of all eruptions that have been suppressed by any means whether external or internal.

Varicose veins of the legs and the thighs.

Varicose veins of pregnancy which have the characteristic of being **painful**.

Burning pain of wounds.

The back of the neck, or waist, tired from writing or typing. The child can only see objects by looking at them from the side. He hates anybody to touch his back.

Agitation of the legs and the feet: **the syndrome of legs that are restless**, like *Tarentula, Rhus tox.*, and *Causticum*.

Sweating of the feet with excoriation between the toes.

Aggravation especially at night, in the evening, and during menses. **Haemoptysis before and during menses**.

This remedy has a very special kind of pruritus. It is **pruritus of the popliteal spaces,** with or without lesion. Eczema, especially behind the ears.

Very sensitive to noise, even the sound of voices.

The child repeats everything said to him before replying.

Forehead cold, occiput hot.

Cross-eyed, rolls the eyes.

Pruritus, especially of the inner canthus.

Pain of the face in general and during headache.

Can't stand even the slightest bit of wine without headache.

A curious, but precious symptom:cannot urinate except sitting down or leaning backwards.

Involuntary urination on walking, coughing, or sneezing.

Pupils who constantly move their legs to stop themselves from urinating and get scolded by the teacher.

Sudden hunger at 11 o'clock in the morning.

Pain in the left ovary.

The child holds the genitals while coughing.

Lienteric stools.

Gas during stool.

Delicate skin, hypersensitive to the least friction and even to the rubbing of garments, must wear silk underwear to avoid irritation.

Nerium oleander: As you know, this is often used as decoration and we find it growing in large pots in outdoor cafés, with its pretty pink or white flowers.

It acts on the nervous system and brings about, first of all, painless paralysis. It acts on the heart bringing about anxious and violent palpitations. It acts on the skin bringing about **pruritus of the scalp day and night**, better from scratching.

It also has an eruption with gnawing pain after scratching.

Like *Paris quadrifolia*, it has the **feeling that the eyes are pulled back into the head**.

It is a vesicular remedy; eczematous and herpetic lesions. All the eruptions of *Oleander* are **prurient and bleed and suppurate on scratching.**

It has a very particular pulse, which I have already spoken about: **an arrhythmic and myurous pulse** (like a rat's tail!)

Extreme weakness of the digestive tract.

REACTIVE REMEDIES OF DIGESTIVE STATES

Phosphoric acid:Is a remedy of weakness, lack of vitality.

Growing children who are always tired. Those lanky fellows like string beans who are always exhausted and don't do any work at school.

Rings around the eyes.

Mydriasis.

Exhaustion.

Nervous sometimes from physical or mental overwork.

Onanists, who continually feel guilty.

Indicated after many acute illnesses which have followed each other in rapid succession; loss of vital fluid or after breast-feeding.

Health affected by **breast-feeding which exhausts**.

After excesses, sorrows, disappointed love, homesickness.

Apathy, and indifference.

Fermentative dyspepsia.

Bites his tongue, especially at night, during sleep.

Frequent diarrhoea, which does not exhaust. He is tired from everything, but not from having diarrhoea!

Always picking his nose.

Occipital headache.

Nicturia; phosphaturia.

Stumbles when walking.

Great desire for fruits, juicy things, and cold drinks.

Thirst for cold milk, like *Phosphorus* and *Tuberculinum*.

Neuritic pains in ghost limbs, after amputation

Relieves the pains of Cancer.

Hair prematurely gray.

NOSODES

I already mentioned the principal indication of the Nosodes: when a case does not make any more progress after a first improvement you can give the patient a Nosode to bring about a reaction. And if the Nosode benefits the patient you may continue it: this is in contrast to the other so-called reactive remedies, which one will not continue in these circumstances.

Just to remind you, a Nosode is "a medicine derived from pathological tissues or secretions containing the specific virus of the sickness"

Psorinum: You know that *Psorinum* is the chronic of *Sulphur*. This is a **very chilly remedy**, even in summer. This is also the patient who is dirty and smells bad: even if he washes himself he always **smells bad**. All the secretions and discharges are very malodorous.

These patients are always **hungry** and, curiously, **especially at night**. They will even get up at night to go out and eat. This is very bad for them, because we know that stomach cancer tends to develop in people who can't stop eating.

Psorinum has a particular pruritus which is an indication and a precious one: **pruritus of the external auditory duct**.

It is also a very good remedy for constipation in children.

Keynote: feels particularly good the day before falling ill.

Tuberculinum bovinum: As I have often said, this is **the only** tuberculin, with *Avicular tuberculin* and *Bacillinum*, **which has been proven on healthy men.** As for the other tuberculins, the indications we have are theoretical, arbitrary, conventional, and empirical. The indications of *Tuberculinum* so readily given, copied, and published by VANNIER are nearly all from NEBEL, and should have been reconsidered, verified, and weighed a long time ago by further provings, I mean by experimentation on healthy man, as in fact any remedy which has the honor of being called homoeopathic should be, and one will never stress this point sufficiently.

I have always given *Tuberculinum bovinum*, when indicated, according to ALLEN and HERING, with excellent results. I cured eruptions, rheumatism, all kinds of cases with this remedy. At the moment I am treating the wife of a homoeopathic doctor from Lyon, and she had been treated by many without any results except a constant and immediate aggravation after all the remedies and nosodes she took. To start the case I gave her one dose of *Tuberculinum*, which 'opened the case' as we say, and which benefited her considerably and immediately.... this reminds me of another patient who came from Patagonia by plane with her husband. She had suffered for years from a sort of mixed eruptions on the face, it was acne form and eczematous, and nobody had been able to do anything for her, and this depressed her morally quite terribly, for she was a pretty woman. I gave her *Tuberculinum bovinum* 10M because she had a little thread in the right eye, indicating a hereditary tuberculinic condition, which was later confirmed by her family history: a paternal uncle (right eye) had been tubercular. And the result was extraordinary: total and permanent cure, after a painful aggravation which lasted two weeks and which she bore with courage.

So this is a remedy which I like particularly, and have no need for any Spengler, Marmorecs, or Denys, etc. ... with their purely theoretical and conventional indications.

It's a wonderful remedy when there is a tubercular heredity, and you can discover this in the eye easily!

Strongly indicated when the symptoms constantly change and the patient catches cold easily.

Emaciation.

This patient loves to travel, journeys and cruises.

He doesn't like standing, like *Sulphur*.

Fear of dogs: very good symptom. I have often told you, when I am consulted for infants who take cold frequently and when I find in the eyes of the mother or the father little indications of tuberculosis, I ask three questions: "What are the animals that your child likes or doesn'tlike? "What are his palms like? "When you scold him what does he do?"

Children who need *Tuberculinum* feardogs;the palms of the hands are damp;when you scold them,even if they are very little,they lift their fists and threaten you back . . . the naughty things!

Here we have some good symptoms:

Likes refined cuisine.

Likes **sweets**.

Likes cold milk.

Likes meat, delicatessen products, ham, lard, smoked meat, but certain subjects have an aversion for meat, for wine, and even for all food.

In contrast to *Tarentula* he has aggravation from music.

And an excellent clinical indication: chronic cystitis (NEBEL).

The pulse is irregular.

Medorrhinum: I am lucky enough to have an excellent source of *Medorrhinum*. A few years ago I was visiting Seville and there I met a charming homoeopathic physician who gave me a quite special gift. You know that Seville is a very pleasant town, full of castanets and pretty women....and also blennorrhagia reigns there as queen! And this doctor had a source taken from a young officer who had goodness knows how many blennorrhagias! He gave me not one drop of pus but a potentisation which he had prepared himself, a fresh preparation which gave me excellent results. First of all and before everything else, it is in no way necessary to have caught blennorrhagia to benefit from this precious Nosode...fortunately!

Patients who need this remedy find that time passes too slowly.

Many of these patients can't speak without weeping; they fear the dark and imagine that there's always someone behind them, and that's why they keep looking back when they walk!

As you may know, there's aggravation especially in the daytime.

It has this very special **sleeping position**; the **genupectoral position.** Thanks to this symptom I cured a case of epiphora, that is, constant watering of the eyes. My patient was a little girl of five or six who had of course been treated without any result by allopathic paediatricians and ophthalmologists who were nevertheless quite reputed... but of course they were allopaths! I don't know if you've ever seen a specialist introducing a catheter into the lachrymal duct of a child; it's quite dreadful. First of all one has to find the orifice and in order to do that you have to put a drop of fluorescein into the eye, and since that burns the child starts kicking, and the fun is on. One really has to have fairy fingers to avoid wounding the eye and causing a retractile scar!

This is where Homoeopathy is marvellous: a well-chosen little remedy and everything proceed smoothly without any dangerous probing. I had given this child several remedies which I had repertorised, but without any result. So I took the father aside and asked him about the illnesses he had had before. That was when he confessed to having had a blennorrhagia in his youth which had been suppressed by the usual injections! After this I learned that the child always slept in this special position: on her knees with her little behind in the air and her head in the pillow, the position which we call the knee-chest position!

Therefore I immediately gave her *Medorrhinum* 10M and since then it was all over... good-bye epiphora! And yet, you know, *Medorrhinum* isn't indicated in the **Repertory** for epiphora. This is one of the wonderful things about Homoeopathy: the remedy that comes up when you repertorise the pathological symptoms isn't always the right one. You sometimes have to work back to the chronic miasm to remove the obstacle. It may be rather difficult to see the relationship between a watering eye and the position in which a patient sleeps.

Women sometimes have a very strange symptom, cold breast and, stranger still, especially the right!

Medorrhinum always feels better at the seaside; better lying on the stomach. Fidgety feet syndrome, especially at night; trembling arms and legs.

There are two more disagreeable symptoms (or agreeable ones, depending on the case):sterility and impotence. This is the great remedy for blennorrhagia suppressed by irrigation or some drug that has stopped the infectious discharge.

In women, intense pruritus of the genitals; very malodorous periods; excoriating leucorrhoea smelling of fish; ovaritis, especially left; sterility; intense dysmenorrhoea.

Chronic catarrh which never ends, especially in children; end of nose always cold; constant desire to be fanned; aphthae.

Monoarticular rheumatism: particularly affecting the knee. Chronic rheumatism. Syndrome of fidgety feet; burning hands and feet, but sometimes cold extremities; trembling arms and legs.

Ferocious appetite, even after having eaten; *Medorrhinum* is always very thirsty; desires liqueurs; desires salt, sweets, warm food; vomiting of pregnancy.

Intense anal pruritus, frequently redness of the anal region in babies.

Nocturnal enuresis.

Finally, intense itching of the skin.

When we study the Nosodes together we shall have to write them into the repertory, because it has only a very small number of indications.

Syphilinum: All symptoms aggravated at night.

These patients are always washing their hands.

A feeling as if the sternum was pulled backwards against the spinal column.

Despair of recovery, like *Calcarea, Arsenicum,* and *Alumina.* Like *Nux vomica,* these patients are completely exhausted in the morning.

Desire for alcoholic beverages.

Erratic rheumatism.

Better in the mountains.

Profuse salivation at night on sleeping, and like *Mercurius* it soils the pillowcase.

When you study your cases you come up with one principal remedy and several satellites: look for the miasm which corresponds to these remedies. If these remedies belong to the three kingdoms, mineral, animal, and vegetable this means that the case is profoundly deep rooted. If there are only mineral remedies this means that it will be a long chronic case and will be difficult to cure. If there are only animal remedies, you can expect complications and difficulties of every kind:this case will be troublesome because of the patient's reactions. And if you have only vegetable remedies it means that the cure will be easy. Find out also if these remedies are exclusively sycotic or psoric or syphilitic. Contrary to what NEBEL believed, **tuberculosis** is not by any means psoro-syphilis, it is **psoro-sycosis**. In the eyes one can also see syphilitic heredity, even several generations back.

Night terrors in infants.

Falling hair.

Patchy alopecia.

Recurrent keratitis.

Although one of the principal indications for Nosodes is an improvement which stops and goes no further (when the therapeutic progression is arrested), one may give them right from the beginning, especially when there is a lack of reaction. As you know these are remedies of an entirely different kind.

Sulphur is a very great reactive remedy but it has the great inconvenience of awakening symptoms just about everywhere and sometimes gives us very disagreeable aggravations; and that is why I haven't mentioned it in the reactive remedies. Still, it is one of our best reactive remedies. Of course one will think of giving it after some other remedies which already have brought some improvement; as a general rule avoid giving it at the beginning of a case.

When you have a defective case, think also of going back to earlier symptoms from the beginning of the illness, old symptoms on which you will be able to prescribe the remedy which the patient should have had before; that remedy can still help him.

After having studied the reactive remedies we should read what HAHNEMANN has to say in Paragraph 184 of his **Organon**."In like manner, after each new dose of medicine has exhausted its action, when it is no longer suitable and helpful, the state of the disease that still remains is to be noted anew with respect to its remaining symptoms, and another homoeopathic remedy sought for, as suitable as possible for the group of symptoms now observed, and so on until the recovery is complete".

Of course, this means questioning your patient again. If you don't know which remedy to give, don't hesitate to give Saccharum lactis. **Do not give a remedy if you have no clear indication**. You will never regret having given Sac lac., but you will always regret having given something which will have upset your case.

I have already told you how Dr. MATTOLI used to manage his practice at the beginning of the vacation period. You know that he was a very short man. He used to dress all in white and in July received his patients not in Florence where he lived, but in Viareggio, in an enormous and magnificent property. That is where he invited my wife and me one summer. For ten days he served us chicken every day! The chicken was exquisite because each time it was differently cooked. One day he prepared polenta on an enormous marble table; it was very amusing. Well, on one occasion the chicken wasn't cooked exactly as he wanted it, and he went to the kitchen. We heard dreadful screams. He slapped the servant in the kitchen a couple of times (and even rather more than a couple of times) - as that was the way he did things - and then he came back to us, much calmed down and quite happy; and we were able to eat our chicken ... in peace!

"When it is time to go on vacation", he used to say, "one is overworked, a great many people keep telephoning, one is harassed and makes wrong prescriptions."

And so, to avoid prescribing wrongly, he used to sit out in the country under a wonderful oak tree, with his secretary at his right hand, and all his case histories. People used to come on horseback, on foot, on bicycles, in motor cars, in carriages... it looked like a camp that had been set up. There must have been at least 200 people! And so Dr. MATTOLI received them under his tree one after the other, and each one of them asked for a remedy for an uncle or an aunt or the cook or the dog or the cat as well - it was dreadful! I can tell you that he didn't waste any time and didn't ask anybody to do a complete strip-tease to auscultate them! But everything worked out very well with the heat of summer and the volubility of the beautiful Italian language! Next to him there was cupboard of remedies, and our colleague prescribed for everybody *Sac lac*... And he had noticed that with the help of the holidays there were hardly 10 percent of the patients who were not much improved when he returned in autumn. Naturally, serious cases didn't come to the country to see him! Fortunately!

Paragraph 185: "Among the one-sided diseases an important place is occupied by the so-called **local maladies**, by which term is signified those changes and ailments that appear on the external parts of the body. Till now the idea prevalent in the schools was that these parts were alone morbidly affected, and that the rest of the body did not participate in the disease - a theoretical, absurd doctrine - which has led to the most disastrous medical treatment".

Paragraph 186: "Those so-called local maladies which have been produced a short time previously, solely by an external lesion; still appear at first sight to deserve the name of local diseases. But then the lesion must be very trivial, and in that case it would be of no great moment. For in the case of injuries accruing to the body from without, if they are at all severe, the whole living organism sympathizes; there occur fever, etc.

"The treatment of such diseases is relegated to surgery; but this is right only in so far as the affected parts require mechanical aid, whereby the external obstacles to the cure, which can only be expected to take place by the agency of the Vital Force, may be removed by mechanical means e.g.:

"By the reduction of dislocations:

"By needles and bandages to bring together the lips of wounds;

"By mechanical pressure to still the flow of blood from open arteries;

"By the extraction of foreign bodies that have penetrated into the living parts;

"By making an opening into a cavity of the body in order to remove an irritating substance or to procure the evacuation of effusions or collections of fluids;

"By bringing into apposition the broken extremities of a fractured bone and retaining them in exact contact by an appropriate bandage, etc.

"But when in such injuries the whole living organism requires, **as it always does, active dynamic aid** to put it in a position to accomplish the work of healing, e.g. when the violent fever resulting from extensive contusions, lacerated muscles, tendons and blood vessels requires to be removed by medicine given internally, or when the external pain of scalded or burnt parts needs to be homoeopathically subdued, then the services of the dynamic physician and his helpful Homoeopathy come into requisition".

Apropos of the Vital Force, KENT mentions these illnesses which are not local (as they are wrongly called), but, instead, **localized illnesses**: when it is an illness that is not surgical, when you have, for instance, an eruption or a small tumor somewhere.

Paragraph 187: "But those affections, alterations and ailments appearing on the external parts that do not arise from any external injury or that have only some slight external wound for their immediate exciting cause, are produced in quite another manner; their source lies in some internal malady. To consider them as mere local affections, and at the same time to treat them only, or almost only, as it were surgically, with topical application or other similar remedies - as the old school have done from the remotest ages - is as absurd as it is pernicious in its results."

For instance, traumatisms often quite benign can be the cause of Osteosarcomas or Carcinomas, which appear years later.

Paragraph 188: "These affections were considered to be merely topical, and were therefore called **local diseases**, as if they were maladies exclusively limited to those parts wherein the organism took little or no part, or affections of these particular visible parts of which the rest of the living organism, so to speak, knew nothing."[4]

Of course, HAHNEMANN was not very tender ... but people were even less tender toward him; and I find that he was even modest in his remarks!

Paragraph 189: "And yet very little reflection will suffice to convince us that no external malady (not occasioned by some important injury from without) can arise, persist or even grow worse without some internal cause, without the cooperation of the whole organism, which must consequently be in a diseased state. It could not make its appearance at all without the consent of the whole of the rest of the health, and without the participation of the rest of the living whole (of the Vital Force that pervades all the other sensitive and irritable parts of the organism); indeed, it is impossible to conceive its production without the instrumentality of the whole (deranged) life; so intimately are all parts of the organism connected together to form an individual whole in sensations and functions. No eruption on the lips, no whitlow can occur without previous and simultaneous internal ill-health".

Except for these traumas, there are therefore no local illnesses. There are only the localized illnesses of a general state of health that is deficient.

There are things which we cannot understand. How can one have, for instance, eczema of the foot and a wart on the ear and strabismus all at the same time? We cannot see at all the connection between these three things and yet they are connected by some biological unity. And that is why we have to base our decisions on the **totality of the symptoms** in choosing a remedy. And even if we don't know the relationship which unites these different morbific complaints, it exists nonetheless; and it is the **fundamental unity** that is reached by our constitutional remedy.

It is very important to meditate upon these paragraphs.

These illnesses are defective; they are partial illnesses, localized illnesses, which we call apparently local. To mention a few of these, we have:

Surgical affections which can be treated by Homoeopathy: I mean, one should always treat the patient before an operation. And we see, if we are good prescribers like Dr. WARD, of San Francisco, famous for his excellent work **Unabridged Dictionary of the Sensations 'As if'**, that a certain number of operations can thus be avoided. Dr. WARD was a Surgeon, a Gynaecologist, who became interested in Homoeopathy, and stated at the end of his life that 40 percent of the patients who came for an operation no longer needed to have that operation after they had been prepared for the operation homoeopathically! In addition, his colleagues were jealous of him and couldn't understand why his operations were more successful. When one can prepare a patient who must undergo a surgical operation, there are two things to which I always call people's attention. First of all, I take the biological rhythms of FLIESS into account to determine the most favourable **date** for the operation. In this way I avoid a great many postoperative complications.

Recently a patient whom I was treating for his general health and who lives in Ungerdien came to see me to ask about having a hernia operation. This was a perfectly straight forward inguinal hernia. I calculated his biological rhythms and advised him about a suitable date. Naturally, surgeons have a thousand and one reasons for not doing what one asks them to do. This patient's surgeon couldn't operate on him on the date he requested and started laughing at him when he spoke about biological rhythms! He operated outside of the good dates. Of course, the operation was very successful, but on the seventh day after the operation the patient felt a pain half way up the inner surface of the thigh as if he were being poked by a red-hot iron every time he stood up. And the surgeon whom he had consulted came and said to him: "Listen, here, sir, this is none of my business. We operated on your hernia and everything went well. Your testicles are not swollen, and you ought to be grateful because that often happens. The trouble you have there is neuralgia and you had better see your doctor about it!" So the patient telephoned to me and asked me what he should do ...and I was very annoyed. He wanted to come to Geneva, but it was quite impossible for him to get into a taxi because the pain was so intense! Naturally, when one doesn't see the patient one cannot always think of everything. Nevertheless, I blame myself for not having been more thoughtful because, after all, after a hernia operation one can easily have reactions of the testicle, and other reactions, too, which are well known.

Neither rest, nor the anticoagulants administered had the slightest effect on the distorting pain felt as soon as he sat down.

We are surprised to discover that it is almost intolerable not to be able to sit down!You can't, after all, remain standing or walking all the time!What a benediction it is to be able to sit down! May be you have never thought about it... Well, finally, the worried surgeon told him to go to see a doctor because it was none of his business! And this went on for three weeks!

I encouraged the patient to try to come to Geneva, but this meant six hours in the train with no hope of sitting down... how happy that was! When he arrived in Geneva, I administered a few points of Acupuncture, which relieved him a little. I gave him first of all *Hypericum* 10M, and two days after discovering that this was in fact a neuralgia of the spermatic duct, a funiculalgia, *Hamamelis* 200 (page 702 of the repertory) every 6 hours for two days. This cured him completely and permanently.

I really think that if one takes into account the rhythms of FLIESS one can avoid a lot of trouble. For instance in blood transfusions, I am thinking of a colleague from Zurich, a great specialist of transfusions, who one day had to give his wife a blood transfusion: well, although he was nearly always successful, this time his wife had an embolism.... and died! He had operated on her on a day when her three rhythms changed simultaneously.

CARLETON, an American, has published a book which I recommend to you, called **Homoeopathy and Surgery**. He was a pure homoeopath and an excellent surgeon, and in this book he gives excellent advise on the homoeopathic treatment of many surgical cases.

In sprains, after manipulation, when this is necessary, Homoeopathy offers a whole palette of very precious remedies which considerably shorten the convalescence and ease the pains. Distensions of the muscles or the tendons of the hand or foot, with or without injury of the periosteum and the bones, can be relieved and often cured in record time after putting them back in position by rubbing with oil of *Rhus* or tincture of *Arnica* and bandaging tightly; after this, one should administer a so-called trauma remedy.

In the **Repertory** on page 1371 you will find remedies for all kinds of distensions of the ligaments, sprains, luxations... etc... in the rubric "Lifting, straining of muscles and tendons."and you can very easily combine this rubric with "Pain, as if sprained" you can add the following remedies: **Arn.**, *Bell-p.*, **Led.**, **Mill.**, **Ruta**, *Agn-c.*, *Am-c.*, *Asaf.*, *Carb-an.*

Under "sprained" you can add "chronic", when the complaint becomes chronic: there is a remarkable remedy indicated by HERING which I have often verified, and that is *Stront-carb*. The 10M potency works beautifully!

On page 983 you have "Dislocation": spontaneous, of the hip: of the kneecap; of the ankle.

If there is weakness of the ligaments look at page 1232 "Weakness, ankle, while walking". And you can add to that rubric *Calc-p.* For children who are late in learning to walk": *Carb-an.*

On page 364 you will find spontaneous dislocation of the jawbone ("Dislocation of jaws easy"), and add to that rubric *Caust,* and *Petr.*

On page 1019 under "Injuries, hand, sprain" you can add *Bell-p.*

Where we have fractures of course we have to

assure the mechanical replacement of fractured bones. But after this, homoeopathic remedies considerably aid osteogenesis and shorten the time of knitting. Usually I give all my patients with fractures *Symphytum* 30 liquid, six drops three times a day for a month, if there are no other personal symptoms. You will find fractures on page 1402 under "Slow repair of broken bones". On page 1008 you can add the rubric "Fractures" Just before "Freezing", with the following remedies: Calc., **calc-p**., calen., **ruta**, *sil.,* **symph**., and under the following rubric: "Consolidation retarded": *ferr.,*

On page 1402 "Slow repair" add *Calen., ferr.*, iod., mang-ac., *mez.*, **Ruta., Symph**. and *thyr.* (CLARKE)

If we have retarded ossification in children think of *Calc., calc-f., Calc-p.*, and *sil.*

Come back to page 1008 and add under "Fractures": (HERING)

"of cranium": *calen*

"infected, with suppuration": **arn**.

"open": *calen.*

"of tibia": *anthr.*

On page 1368 you will find the rubric "Injuries", which includes blows, falls, ecchymoses ... etc. Add Acet-ac., acon., ang., bufo, *calen., camph.*, crot-t., glon., ham., mag-c., *mill.,* phys., *stront-c.,* verb., and on the following page under the rubric "with extravasations" add *led.*

Forinsomnia after fractures or after surgery think of *stict.*

For contusions of the nerves, on page 1369, add bell-p.,

For contusions of soft parts add *ham.*, and *symph.*

In contusions of the tendons add calen.

BOERICKE indicates for contusions: acet-ac., **arn**., bell-p., *con*., echi., euphr., *ham*., *hyper*., led., *rhus-t*., ruta, sul-ac., symph., and verb.

And for the chronic results of traumatisms: **arn**., carb-v., cic., *con*., glon., ham., hyper., led., *nat-s*., *stront-carb.*

On the last page of the **Repertory**, page 1422, you have the whole question of 'wounds'; under this rubric you can add 'lacerated': arn., *calen*., **carb-ac**., ham., *hyper*., led., staph., sul-ac., symph.(BOERICKE).

Under the general rubric "wounds" add *calen*., carb-ac., helianathus,(CLARKE).

Under "bites" add: Lob-pur., and *Seneg.*

"snakes": thuj.;

"bleeding freely": am-c., dor., ham., **lat-m., nit-ac.,** ph-ac., **sanguisuga.**

"crushed": *carb-ac., ruta*;

"cuts": calen, ham., hyper,;

"decubitus, see sore": *all-c., tub*,;

"gangrene, tendency": calen., sal-ac., sul-ac., (BOERICKE);

"painful" *all-c.*;

"penetrating": phaseolus;

"painful injections": crot-h., led,;

"to remove thorns, splinters, fishbones": *lob., sil.*;

"proud flesh": sil.;

"if the injured part feels cold to the patient and to objective touch": *led*.

Under "Burns", page 1346, add acet-ac,. acon., arn., calc-p., calen., camph., gaultheria., grin., ham., *hep*., jab., *kali-bi*., kreos., ter., urt-u.;

"burns from X-rays": calc-f., x-ray;

"burns fail to heal, or ill effects": carb-ac., caust.

On page 1304 you will find something which may often help you, "cicatrices". For keloids you will combine the two rubrics "elevated" and "hard". In the rubric "hard" you should put **graph.**, into the third degree and add *fl-ac.* CLARKE recommends an ointment with *Staphysagria* in the mother tincture.

For keloid scars there is whole series of remedies to be added. I found them during my searches in the works of the great ALLEN, BOERICKE, CLARKE, JAHR, LILIENTHAL, STAUFFER, and DOUGLAS: ars., bell-p., calc., carb-v., caust., crot-h., *fl-ac.*, **graph.**, hyper., iod., junc., lach., merc., nit-ac., nux v., ophiotoxicon (JAHR), phos., phyt., psor., rhus-t., sabin., *sil.*, sulph., sul-ac., thios., tub., vipera.

I gave you some examples of so-called localised affections, and now we shall see how to find the remedy in defective illnesses. You have a patient who comes to consult you complaining of only one symptom, or of very vague problems; what are you going to do in such a case and how are you going to find a remedy which can help him?

First of all, before looking for a remedy one should always start by eliminating any habits or extraneous circumstances which might be the cause of the patient's disorder, as HAHNEMANN said at the beginning of his **Organon**.

Here are some guidelines which we must bear in mind for every illness:

1. One must correct the diet. CARTON was right to insist on this point, for it can bring considerable improvement to patients. It is dreadful to see the

diet which some people follow. This reminds me of a certain patient who always keeps a magnificent box of chocolates just inside of his front door: he offers some to anybody who comes to see him and this gives him an opportunity to have some also. One of my women patients, whom I sent to see one day for influenza, had one kilo of candy next to her bed, and from it she would serve herself generously during the night whenever she woke up. She was surprised that she was overweight and that she always had liver trouble!

2. One has to pay attention to the way patients live, their hygiene and their exercise. Advise them to do fifteen minutes of exercise every morning: generally they never do it! A good idea is to have them take lessons in physical exercise from some teacher whom they have to pay. There are stationary cycling and rowing apparatuses which people buy to use at home, and never use for more than one month after buying them at considerable expense! Tell them to take lessons in riding, or tennis, or gymnastics. Then there are also those patients who never take holidays, and for whom the only thing that counts is their work. If you can't get them to take holidays like everybody else, tell them to go on a cruise, or propose some hydro-mineral cure which is as harmless as possible, and which will oblige them to some sort of regular schedule and rest for at least a month. Then of course there are fasts, which can be prescribed for those who can stand them.

3. Examine the spine, and if necessary send the patient to a chiropractor for any necessary adjustments. This is very useful sometimes, and one shouldn't neglect it.

4. Don't forget the dentist. There are people who never go to the dentist. Look at your patients' teeth, carefully sound them, apply heat or cold with a moist wad of gauze. You may find people with unbelievable things in their mouths. I will never forget a certain society lady who had twenty seven of her thirty-two teeth absolutely bathed in pus! And she didn't feel a thing. She had to have all her teeth out, and now she's quite well.

5. Examine the ears. You would be surprised to know how many people go around with plugs of wax as hard as wood in their ears, and how grateful they are when you clean out the ears!

6. Habits. Some people have dreadful habits: some people wear the same clothes for at least twenty years - what a shame! – for instance, a dirty old jacket, all worn-out, or a venerable raincoat. Disgusting! Get them to buy new clothes, and something in their manner changes immediately. In the apartment get them to change the position of the furniture or to swap rooms, or to change pictures on the walls, and their whole condition might change! Especially when there has been some mourning in the family, get them to change the position of the furniture: in this

way the 'perpetual presence'(and sometimes the very trying presence) of the dear departed is dissipated.

Only after all these steps you can start asking yourself what remedy you are going to prescribe. And this is difficult when there are almost no symptoms. When we have what we call a deficient illness you have to have some imagination to see what can be done.

1. The first thing to look for is the etiological symptoms: "ailments from ...": anger (p.2), anticipation (p.4), contradiction (pp.2/512), egotism (p.39), emotional excitement (p.40), fright (p.49), grief (p.51), homesickness (p.51), wounded honor (p.52),indignation (p.55), disappointed love (p.63), reproaches (p.71), rudeness (p.75), scorn (p.78), thinking of complaints (p.87), vexation (p.21), mental work (p.95)

2. You can also find very good information in the hereditary symptoms:those that come from the mother to a boy, from the father to a girl. Take into account also the particular symptoms manifested by the mother during her pregnancy, and during her labor.

3. All suppressions must be noted. Cutaneous affections, discharges; leucorrhea, gonorrhea, sweat, coryza, etc. For the result of polypharmaceutic practices; even before you think of any other remedy you can always give them *Nux vomica*.

4. Vaccinations which either didn't take, or did take. If there was a reaction and it was too strong, this is a good point to start from in prescribing remedies of Vaccinosis, p.1410. If the vaccination didn't take, it means that the individual was either too weak to react, or that the vaccination was no good.
5. Childhood diseases. What interests us particularly are affections of childhood which left after-effects: the child didn't recover quickly, the cure was not clear-cut. Some of them cough for a year or two after whooping cough, and others have endless eye trouble after the measles. We know that scarlatina and mumps can leave consequences and continue to act on the general condition in a dreadful way. The same applies to chicken pox and diphtheria. In these cases think of giving a Nosode which corresponds to the illness, either in the 30th, 200th, or, better, in the 10M potency.
6. There are rubrics which are absolutely objective:the rubric "Old people" - consult it if your patient is more than 60; the rubric "infants" which is not in the present **Repertory** but was in the first edition, and which I have advised you to add to the present edition; the rubrics for nursing mothers and pregnant women.
7. Observe the periodicity.
8. Observe any obesity, thinness, or varicose veins.

You can find these manifestations in the **Repertory** and they can help you a great deal.

We can't find very much under **general symptoms** in defective illnesses. The patient will complain of weakness, general tiredness, without being precise. If the symptoms are there, think especially of seeking out and noting chilliness or warm-bloodedness, and any reactions to extremes of temperature.

As for **mental symptoms**, here again you won't find much, unless this illness is defective only because the doctor is! We are in the habit of asking a great many questions, but, in addition, there are a multitude of little things which we forget because we can't keep everything in our minds—especially if we are defective doctors! Which are the mental symptoms we haven't thought about? We can have a patient who has no fears or anxieties at present, but who may have had some in his youth. Quite often we forget these; for example, fear of solitude, of darkness, of robbers, of storms, of water, of animals. Remember that the individual is, after all, a biological unity.

Often we forget to find out whether our patients were somnambulists during their youth.

Now, concerning ideas of suicide, this is a touchy subject. One should try first of all to bring up the subject indirectly: "In certain difficult moments of life there are people who ....", and from the corner of your eye you can look at your patient to see if he reacts. And if they come to talk to you about wanting to commit suicide, they are reassured just from this little remark. Don't forget also that the flattening of the pupil at twelve o'clock is an indication of this.

You can see so many things. For instance, if the patient starts when the telephone rings, or when a door suddenly slams.

Always find out about weeping: involuntary weeping, uncontrollable weeping, weeping during sleep, etc. And ask them also whether they feel better or worse from it.

Then there is the question of vertigo, which can give us very precise indications when we know how to ask the right questions. For instance, if our patient has vertigo while walking we should find out in which direction he feels pulled: forward, backwards, sideways (and if so, to which side). Always ask whether the vertigo disappears when he closes his eyes. Then there are vertigos which rotate, or vertigos which give the feeling of being pressed under, or of swaying, vertigos with headaches, or with dimness of vision, vertigos from heights, vertigos looking upwards, lifting the head, vertigos looking at objects which move, for instance, cars in the street.

Now, as for the head, you know that Dr. TYLER had a particular predilection for headaches. She said that this was her favourite rubric in all the **Repertory**. It is true that this is the chapter which is most carefully elaborated in its modalities and pains. As a rule patients have great difficulty telling you the kind of pain they feel.

But don't let us forget to ask how the pains appear: do they appear and disappear quickly or gradually? You will find this information on page 141, "increasing gradually"; page 149, "sudden pains"; page 151, "waves of pain".

Ask them also about spots before the eyes, which are a frequent and precious indication of *Iris versicolor* in headaches.

There are also headaches with constipation (p.138) or with colds (p.138). The feeling that the head is empty or full can sometimes help one. Ask them also about the extension of the pains.

One forgets sometimes perspiration of the head, its locality and modality. Sometimes they perspire all over the body and not on the head.

Some people have sensitivity of the scalp from brushing or combing the hair; others can't stand the warmth of a hat (p.121, carb-an., *iod., led., lyc.*,), or on the contrary, can't go without one (p.233, "uncovering")

On page 229 you will find the rubric "Sensitiveness of brain", you should add: "even to hat", *bry., carb-v.*, chin., crot-t., hep., merc., mez., **nit-ac., sil**,staph., sulph. Some people cannot stand pressure, for instance, the weight of a hat, and this corresponds to mez. and nit-ac. according to GENTRY. Under this rubric "Sensitiveness from brushing the hair" you may add Viburnum.

There are patients who have constant headaches, they never stop: and there are two rubrics: "chronic" headaches, (am-c., *ars.*, *caust.*, con., *sil.*, *sulph.*, ter., tub.) and constant continued" headaches, on pages 137 and 138 respectively. For this kind of headache there is a Nosode which you may think of and which may help you very much: *Meningococcinum*. On page 139 you have headaches after haircuts (**bell.**, glon., led., puls., sabad., *sep.*), and on page 151 "pain from washing head". There are also dreadful headaches, badly described, which are often rheumatic headaches (p.146). Then there are wandering headaches or headaches in spots. (p.148)

People never have enough time to examine the eyes thoroughly. But they reveal useful symptoms which the patient will not always tell you.

Eyes which are glued closed in the mornings.

Accumulation of eye gum in the corners of the eyes.

Cracks and fissures. Look for them on the face. You may find them in the outer canthi of the eyes, of the mouth, of the nose. Sometimes they are uricemic. Make your patients sweat, make them take exercise, change their diet, and quite often these little crevices will disappear. There are little cracks on the corners of the nostrils (p. 329, "Cracks"), and at the insertion of the ear (p.288, "Eruptions behind the ears").

The pupils: see their degree of dilation or contraction; anisochorea. Unequal pupils often indicate vago-sympathetic disturbance.

Blepharo-spasms. In the **Repertory** there are three terms which are rather alike. Usually these patients are too tense. They need holidays and rest. In the **Repertory** look under "Quivering" on page 264, "Twitching", and "Winking". A remedy which has often brought me success and which you can add under "Quivering of lids" is *Aranea scinencia*. PATERSON's *Dys-co.* often succeeds also.

Convergent or divergent strabismus.

Chalazions: look to see if they are on the upper or lower lid. The location can help you.

Swelling of the eyes: upper lid or lower lid, or beneath lower lid. Sometimes there is a little swelling of the inner corner above the upper lid, and this can be a sign of hernia. It is also often a typical symptom of *Kali carb*. (p.355, "Bloated, between lids and eye brows").

Cold tears, burning or salty tears.

Hemeralopia.

Disturbances of refraction; you know for instance that a typical remedy for astigmatism is *Tuberculinum*.

Marginal blepharitis is often well taken care of by *Bacillinum* 30 once a week.

Falling eyelashes and eyebrows.

Look at the conjunctiva, whether they are red, pale, or yellowish. Sometimes they will indicate little attacks of jaundice: in that case look also at the palms and the palate to see if they are yellowish.

Some patients constantly rub their eyes (p.265), and this must not be confused with those who **wipe** their eyes (p.270).

Nystagmus: find out whether it is horizontal or rotary.

The **ears**: Sometimes when you look at your patients' ears you see that there is cotton-wool in them and you ask why. "Well it's because I can't stand cold air!"And then you have the remedies for this little symptom: **Acon**., clem., *hep., lac-c.*, merc., *sil., thuj.*

Some people don't know that they had bad hearing in one ear. Similarly some people don't know that they see poorly in one eye; it is up to you to verify these matters.

Always ask your patients if they can perceive the direction from which sounds come: you know that *Carbo animalis* is the great remedy for those who don't know where the sound is coming from.

Others don't hear anything at all when many people are speaking at once: there are even people who hear better in a noise!

The **nose**: The nose also can be very sensitive to the intake of air. There are people who are always picking their nose, and it is often a symptom of worms. Also it may be the sign of a frustrated libido.

As for colds (which doctors fear, because they don't know what to give!), Homoeopathy often succeeds admirably. One could say that eighty percent of the patients who have a cold are immediately improved with *Aconite* 200. We are more interested in obstructions than in discharges, and, in that connection, there are some questions which one would do well to ask properly: On what side? Day or night? In a cold or in a warm atmosphere?

Sometimes it is obstructed and it runs at the same time.

There is a special rubric for obstructed nose in children, and it has excellent remedies: Am-c., *ars.*, asc-t., and for nursing babies: *aur.*, *kali-bi.*, **lyc.**, **nux-v.**, samb. (see NOSE, obstruction p 341)

Dry noses are generally hard to cure.

As for epistaxis, CLARKE highly recommends *Ferrum picricum*: he says this remedy succeeds better than all the others. *Viper* also often succeeds very well for nose bleeds, especially if the blood is dark. There is also a rubric for epistaxis in infants, and the remedy which succeeds most often is *Ferrum phos.* (Abrot., bell., chin-s., *croc.*, *ferr.*, *ferr-p.*, *ferr-pic.*, *ham.*, merc., phos., ter.). Think also of epistaxis at night, washing the face, and all the other possible modalities for which there are specific remedies.

Ask your patient about his sense of smell. Then again sneezing is very important in finding the remedy, and don't forget the modalities. You remember the morning sneezes which is a very good symptom of *Ammonium carbonicum.*

Face: We already spoke of chapped skin, cracked skin, excoriations. Cracks in the upper lip will make you think especially of *Kali carb.* and *Natrum mur.* If there are cracks in the corner of the mouth there are a whole series of remedies: this is the famous angular cheilitis, or commissural ulceration, which is often a sign of a lack of vitamin B2.

The tongue can also have fissures, especially on the sides, and in the middle, and on the tip.

Always look at the complexion, the colour of the face; and look also at the expression. In the **Repertory** there is a rubric which gives very detailed attention to the expressions of the face: surprised, anxious, worried, aged, tired, sickly expression, etc. Sometimes these signs will help you to find the remedy. Look also at the wrinkles and the frowns. They may be important.

The perspiration of the face may be hot or cold, or may appear only on one side, or on the upper or lower lip etc. Some people only perspire on the nose (and of course the classic remedy is *Tuberculinum bov.*)

Mouth: Sometimes the aphthae in the mouth are very troublesome: sometimes also the fault lies with the dentist with his little wads of cotton powdered with Borax. Look at the location of these aphthae: they may be on the gums, on the tongue, or on the lips. You might try a little mouth-wash with lemon juice: it hurts at first, but sometimes it feels much better afterwards. My professor of ophthalmodiagnosis had another method: he used to use a little wad of gauze saturated with an infusion of chamomilla, with which he scraped the aphthae until they bled... and that was that. On page 397 you will find aphthae of the mouth, and in the general rubric you might add: Sempervivum tectorum (Houseleek). And also, cinch-b., ill., ip., while phos., sars., and semp; should be in italics.

Lower down, under "in children", add bapt., asim., kali-br., plant., viol-t. Add "in infancy": bry.; and "in influenza": ant. t.

Think of Kali mur. when the aphthae progress towards ulceration;

And for aphthae of the lips: cadm., cinch-b., cub., ip., jug-r., kali-c., mur-ac., hep., **Merc-c**.

For aphthae of the palate add: Sempervivum, sul-ac., and underline phos.

Look at the tongue, whether it is dry or wet., whether it oscillates or trembles.

Among the different smells of the breath there is one so disagreeable that we call it 'sickening': it makes you sick if you have to be subjected to it! In such cases, before thinking of a remedy, you might advise the patient to buy a tongue rake, and to use a mouth-wash of calendula lotion after it.

Some patients sleep with the mouth open (p. 409).

On page 417 you have the rubric "Salivation". In the main rubric delete calad; and add: aur., calc-ars., eucal., hipp., merc-sol., nit-s-d., phys., squil., ter., ust., verat-v., vinc. xanth.

Under "Salivation" add the following rubrics and remedies:

"night": culex, merc-c.

"acrid": lact., merc.

"angina, in": bar-m.

"aphthae, with": bell., **Merc**. **Merc-c**., nat-m.

"apoplexia, in": anac. **Nux v**.

"asthma, in": carb-v.

"cardialgia, in": puls.

Children": camph.

"chill and fever, with": stram.

"coryza with": calc-p. cupr-a.

"dentition, in": hell., merc-sol., nat-m., Sil.

"dribbling": stram.

under "dryness, with sense of" add kali-m.

"esquinancia": anthr.

"fetid breath, with": Kali-br.

"fever, during": sulph.

under "headache, during" add cimb.

"measles, in": nat-m.

under "mercury, from" add hydr.

"numps, in": nat-m.

"nausea, with": **Ip**., camph., carb-s., chin., lach., sulph., verat.

under "pregnancy, during" add: ip., **Goss**.

"prosopalgia, in": mez., plat.

"scarlatina, in": **Arum-t**., caps., **Lach**., merc., sulph.

"malignant": **Am-c**.

under "sleep, during" add a note to "(See Night)", and add: cinch-b., dios., ip., and put kali-c., into italics.

"sleep, preventing": ign.

"speaking, constant while": graph., lach.

"spit, with constant desire to": cocc-c., cadm-s., graph., grat., lac-c., lyss., puls.

"swallow, constantly obliged to": ip., seneg.

"toothache, with": **Cham**., daph., kali-m., nat-m., and add a note to ("See Teeth, pain, saliva, with involuntary flow of, p. 438)".

"tonsillitis cough, in": **Bar-c**.

"whooping cough, in": **bry**., **iris-v**., spong.

Then there is "Speech, stammering", page 419, and "Speech, lisping", page 419. Ask about the sense of taste: the loss of taste or different perversions of taste.

Teeth: You have to examine the teeth of your patients: any caries, the color of the teeth, and any deformation; then you have the untidy tooth of Topinard, which of course is none other than the wisdom tooth! From my personal experience, one should always extract a wisdom tooth if it causes trouble or grows wrongly.

Throat: Always look at the condition of the uvula: it hangs like a little sack of water; perhaps there are aphthae on it, or small whitish deposits. One should examine the tonsils also.

Neck: Notice whether your women patients wear a scarf; some of them can't stand having anything round the neck.

Then there is the whole question of goitres: I confess that I have never managed to make goitre disappear. Sometimes my patients have said that they felt much better, but in measuring the neck I noticed that there was no change – it as purely subjective. But after having treated patients with goitre for a certain time for their general condition, you may find that they tolerate an operation on the goitre very well, without any after effects.

Food desires and aversions: From page 480 on you will find all the aversions to food, and you may add the following:

under "cheese" put olnd. into italics and add: arg-n., nit-ac., staph., and add the following sub-rubrics:

"Roquefort": hep.

"strong": hel., nit-ac.

"Swiss (Gruyere)": merc., sulph.

"Chicken": bacillinum (Allen).

under "fruit" add: ars., **Chin.**, **Puls**. carcin., and add the following sub-rubric.

"green": mag-c.

under "milk" add: carcin., **Staph**.

under "onions" add thuj.

under "salt food" add carcin.

"strawberries": chin., sulph.

under "sweets" add nux v., puls.

Under "Desires", from page 483 on, make the following additions:

under "alcoholic drinks" add the following sub-rubric: "habit, to remove": strych-n., 3X

under "beer, evening": add med., and put zinc. into italics.

under "beer" add another sub-rubric:

"thirst, without": calad.

under "chocolate" add: carcin. sep.

"fat food, which aggravates": ars., hep., **Nit-ac**., nux v., sulph., tub., carcin.

under "fat ham" and carcin.

under "indigestible things" add: nit. ac., nux v.

under "lemons" add: bell., nabalus.

under "meat" add the following sub-rubric:

"children, in": mag-c.

under "milk" add carcin.

under "onions, raw" add thuja.

under "salt things" add carcin.

under "sweets" put merc. into italics, and ad under "sugar" the following sub-rubric:

"only digests if he eats large amounts of sugar": nux v., **Staph**.

under "tea" add puls.

under "tobacco" add: med., nicotine, plant, and add the following sub-rubric:

"to remove desire for": calad., calc., **Caust**., ign., lach., nux v., petr., plan., **Staph**., sulph. (Gallavardin).

"tomatoes, raw": ferr.

Desires sweet and sour foods at the same time: bry., calc., carb-v., kali-c., med., sabad., sec., sep., **Sulph**.

Desires sour and salty food: arg-n., calc., calc-s., **Carb-v**., con., **Cor-r**., med., merc-i-f., **Nat-m**., **Phos**., plb., sulph., thuj., **Verat**.

Desires sweets and salt: **Arg-n**., calc., carb-v., med., plb.

Desires sweets, which aggravated: am-c., **Arg-n**., calc., nat-c., **Sulph**.

Stomach: Eructations can help us a great deal: so can yawning and sneezing. Some eructations ameliorated, others aggravated. Ask your patient about the taste of these eructations. You will find all this from page 489 onwards. There are nosy eructations, others that are controlled.

Ask your patient about hiccough, and if he has hiccoughs modalities can be very important. If you make a medical certificate, never mention the word "hiccough", but speak instead "phrenoglottic myoclonias", which makes a very good impression and forces people to look in the dictionary! You will find hiccoughs on page 501, and under the general rubric add: ambr., amyl-n., ars-h., calad., cupr-s., hydr., hydr-ac., med., lyss., sin-n., staph., stront., tarax., and make the following additions:

under "night" add the following sub-rubric:

"urination, with involuntary": hyos.

"apoplexy, in": ol-caj.

"asthma, begins attack of": cupr.

"back, with pain in": teucr.

"carried, when, in cholera infantum": kreos.

"children, in": bor., ign., ip.

"nursing, while", hyos.

"after": teucr.

"restlessness at night, with": stram.

"cholera, in": aeth., arg-n., cic., cupr., mag-p., ph-ac. verat.

"concussion of brain, in": hyos.

under "convulsions, with" put cupr. into italics, and add stram.

under "cough, after" add ang.

"diarrhoea, with": cinnam., verat.

under "dinner, before": put mur-ac. into italics

under "dinner, after" put phos., into italics

under "drinking, after" put puls. into italics

under "eating, after" add: filix-m., ham., and put par. into italics.

"emotions, after": ign.

under "eructations, after" add: ars-h., ox-ac.

under "fever, during" add the following sub-rubric: "yellow, in": ars-h.

"fruits, after cold": ars., puls.

"gastralgia, with": sil.

"gastric affections, in": kali-bi.

"hepatic colic, in": chin.

"hepatitis, in": bell.

"intestinal intussusception, in": plb.

"migraine, in": aeth.

"meningitis, in": arn.

under "painful" add mag-p., and add the following sub-rubric:

"causes crying": bell.

"peritonitis, in": hyos., lyc.

"salivation, with profuse": lob-i.

"sitting up straight": kreos.

under "smoking, while" add: calen., scutell., and put ign. and sang. into italics

"spine, in affections of": stram.

"stomach, in cancer of": carb-an.

under "supper, after" add coca.

"surgery, after": hyos.

under "typhoid, in" add mag-p.

under "vomiting, while" add: bry., jab., jatroph., **Verat.**, and add the following sub-rubrics:

"before": cupr.

"terminates in": jab.

"winter, in": nit-ac.

For slow digestion add the rubric "Slow" on page 526 (and make cross references to "Inactivity" on page 503, and "Disordered" on page 486): aur-m., berb., **Chin.**, corn., corn-f., cycl., eucal., lyc., nuph., nux v., op., par., sabin., sep., **Sil.**, **Tarent.**

cardio-pyloric stenosis: see pages 483, 504, 511.

Section 5: Treasure Works

MISTAKES MADE IN HOMOEOPATHIC TREATMENT

"HOMOEOPATHIC PHYSICIAN"- what meaning should this title convey? The physician who to the complete equipment of his university studies in medicine and surgery, adds also a thorough acquaintance with homoeopathy and puts its principle into practice, only he has the right to the title "homoeopathic physician". He will have made himself especially familiar with the work of Dr. Samuel Hahnemann, founder of homoeopathy, with the Materia Medica, with repertories, and the laws relative to administration of remedies to the sick.

The study of homoeopathy exacts of the neophyte a definite effort; for he must lay aside prejudices acquired during his university studies. But the method of considering any given case proves to be so different from that which he has hitherto known, that he soon sees the importance of this new method. Now he sees in the "case" who come to consults him, not merely diseases which he must diagnose, but individuals sick, for whom he must find the similar remedy for each, individually.

Also, he must avoid routine; he may not remember other cases resembling this one, which he has already treated; he must isolate the distinctive difference in the sick person whom he now consider, must find out his peculiarities, his individual characteristic. This is a theory essentially and indispensably homoeopathic. Among the tangle of symptoms resulting from his examination, he must distinguish with care those which pertain to the sick one himself, as a thinking and suffering human being, because of which he is burdened with illness, from those others which concern only a portion of his physical organism- a single organ, or group of organs.

The practical result is fully inherent in this great secret on nature, discovered by Samuel Hahnemann: To determine the symptoms representative of the Individual himself who is ill; and not make the blunder of noting alarming who symptoms to any organ which is the point of least resistance where the illness finds for itself an exit, through which it utters its cry of pain.

A true homoeopath finds his task to consist first in establishing a therapeutic diagnosis according to the fundamental laws of homoeopathy discovered by Hahnemann and developed by Lippe, Hering, Allen, Kent, Nash and so many others.

This it is which makes homoeopathy a method not to be surpassed, this "therapeutic diagnosis", I may call it, or "homoeopathic diagnosis", which leads to the remedy immediately without waiting for a "morbid diagnosis"; which treats a patient without having to determine his exact sickness! Observe that I say "exact sickness", for such general terms as hysteria, nervousness, rheumatism, dyscrasic or cryptogenic state, idiopathic, and what not-these do not deserve the noble term "diagnosis". This fine and learned terminology readily covers the ignorance of the doctor giving treatment, ignorance not as to his science, but as to the case he deals with- a very different matter.

The word "diagnosis" alone, connotes a pathological diagnosis, with a verdict of morbidity. It is time to show to those who have not yet learned the fact, that there is a far more practical diagnosis: that is, one indicating from the very outset the necessary remedy. This is what Adolf Lippe meant when he said, "Here is a person of the phosphorus type; here, one of the arsenic types; here of Pulsatilla." And he uses the terms consecrated to these meanings by Hahnemann in the Organon, 1811. Kent also tells in his Lectures on Homoeopathic Philosophy, of a patient who asked him: "Doctor, what is the matter with me?" and he replied: "Why, you have Nux vomica," that being his remedy. Whereupon the old man said: "Well, I did think I had some wonderful disease or other!" That is therapeutic, a homoeopathic diagnosis.

I do not enlarge further upon the point; such diagnosis is clearly the first duty of the homoeopathic physician. Frequently it leads to a prompt, mild and permanent improvement, to a cure of the patient.

But we are not at the end of our task; we face two other heavy responsibilities; one of these concerns the patient, and the other, the future of medical science. Upon us rest both of these responsibilities.

As to the patient-our task is not only to relieve, but to CURE. Now, a true cure rests not solely on a disappearance of existing symptoms, but equally on advice given the patient, that he need not again fall into such a state. Such counsels, of hygiene, of directing work and time, of morale, of reading, of the whole attitude, and control of life-these also presuppose a diagnosis. And here, at this point, the disease diagnosis becomes not only serviceable but indispensable to the doctor. (See Kent, Lectures on Homoeopathic Philosophy, 1919, page 143).

The whole idea of diagnosis, in relation to the task of the physician, is it not just the discovery of that famous "causa occasional is" of which Hahnemann wrote in such details? (See Organon, Sections 7, 73, 77, 150.) The homoeopathic doctor must not simply prescribe pills or drops, but he must be a minister of nature, a "naturist" in addition to a symptom, to give them a purpose is, interpretative analysis, covering their last detail, a complete symptomatological examination.

There are homoeopaths, alas! who do not sufficiently examine even their patients, and who thus bring discredit upon the name, and value of the art of medicine called homoeopathic. That certain clever men may omit such a procedure in examination as we have described, and still by a judicious interpretation of symptoms, cure their patient, is of course possible; but certainly such is not a method which could be generalized. Perhaps a few instances may clarify this thought yet further.

1. A young man of eighteen years of age sought consultation regarding frequent attacks of throat angina, which settled as often on the right side as on the left, and followed almost regularly exposure to cold. Painting with various applications and frequent cauterizations and pulverizations in no way affected his condition and he asked my advice. The symptoms, as he gave them to me, pointed explicitly to Tuberculinum or Sulphur. Yet I gave neither of these remedies, because after further questioning I found that he wore thin low shoes and silk stockings, and that he took cold especially after dancing, or when his feet were cold. Accepting some simple hygienic advice, he wore thicker socks, shoes with rubber soles and gaiters in winter and he had no more throat attacks.

   I acknowledge that possibly the remedy, had I given it, would have removed his tendency to throat affections, but it seemed to me wiser to show him the mistake he was making, and to correct his condition by simple hygienic measures. The therapeutic diagnosis was Tuberculinum; the morbid diagnosis was angina from exposure to cold; the prescription was hygienic advice. Result: a cure.

2. A young woman in domestic service, aged twenty, came to consult me regarding rheumatism in the

legs. She had been treated allopathically for three months, but the salicylates given were making her deaf and producing giddiness. She found herself increasingly weak, walking with difficulty, had vague pains and great weakness in the calves of her legs. Questioning led to a clear indication of Lycopodium, but I did not give that until I had completed the full examination. On reaching the throat I found a curious condition of the pharynx: it looked as if painted with a yellow orange varnish! Taking a culture I found a large number of Klebs-Loffler bacilli, of the short type.

Evidently there was here paralytic trouble, sequels of a diphtheria, which had been overlooked apart from a dryness of the throat, the sick girl had not local symptoms. This diagnosis enabled me to take the measures necessary in this disease. Naturally, I made no serum, but for reasons which I need not detail here, I gave one dose of Lycopodium 200, without observing any result in the following fortnight. The throat remained the same; weakness was still there; no improvement was perceptible. Such total failure of reaction to the indicated remedy led me to give her a dose of Diphtherinum 200, to which the condition responded very well.

In Allens Nosodes (1918, page 40) we read with regard to this remedy:

Painless diphtheria. Symptoms almost entirely objective patient too weak to complain. Patient apathetic. Prostration. Highly susceptible to diphtheritic virus. Post-diphtheritic paralysis. Remedy suitable when the most carefully selected remedy fails to relieve or permanently improve.

The girls throat promptly cleared up and resumed its normal aspect; and at the end of a fortnight, another examination showed not a single bacillus. As the weakness remained, I gave another dose of Lycopodium, of which the effect was surprising the patient got up, began to walk and in ten days was able to return to her work.

Wound psorinum or Tuberculinum have had an equally good effect? How could one determine the suitable Nosode in a case which does not react, save only by making a most carefully disease diagnosis?

3. A young man was treated by a homoeopath for a swelling of glands under the jaw. The homoeopathic treatment was changed frequently during several months, but without result. The doctor examined the man's neck each time. Then the patient consulted another physician who found no remarkable signs in his face, head neck and chest, but on examining the spinal column, he found evidence of Potts Disease. The swelling was only a cold abscess arising from the third cervical vertebra. It was tuberculosis of the bones of the spine, causing suppuration which, descending, produced a swelling below the jaw. The patient was given hygienic advice, rest, mountain air, diet

in accordance with the diagnosis, and medicine based on the diagnosis which cured.

4. A patient, fifty-five years of age, was subject to cold in the head, was nervous, and had suffered for six months from sudden attacks of suffocation. He had been treated by various allopathic physicians with numerous anti-spasmodic and vagotonic medicines with no benefit and had deteriorated still further. The patient walked with his head bowed, often belched aloud, spat continually and was afraid to swallow his saliva. Eating was a veritable tragedy for him, for he remembered that his first attack occurred while eating. He refused to take any liquid food, as this upset him more than solids. Finally he gave up his doctors, for they had told him that he was nervous, that he must pull himself together and that he should disregard his attacks. A first examination revealed nothing obviously abnormal. For a time psychotherapy seemed to alleviate his fears. But neither Mephitis, Ignatia nor Lachesis could stop the attacks which, though less frequent, still occurred too often. After taking cold, laryngitis set in, causing a husky voice. The indicated remedies had no effect. According to all homoeopathic principles, the case was incurable. Examination of the larynx showed a paralysis of the right vocal cord and careful examination revealed a thyroid tumour, very hard, and as large as a tangerine, on the right side. This caused the constriction of an important nerve. His loss of weight, age, complexion, and

various symptoms pointed to the fact that this was a case of thyroid cancer, not a mere laryngitis. Unfortunately the patient found homoeopathy too slow, and returned to an allopathic physician. He applied radium needless which reduced the tumour which caused ulceration, and within eight days the patient died under terrible sufferings.

It is clear that the physician must know quite as well WHAT he is treating as WHOM HE IS TREATING. What can be said of those doctors who, not comprehending the case, called it "nerves" and advised the sufferer to pull himself together?.

5. A young man of twenty had been treated for two years by a homoeopath with Aurum, Calcarea, Ignatia, Pulsatilla, etc. He was highly nervous and had frequent attacks of giddiness while working. He became so distressed and depressed as to weep hot tears. He worked in a bank, but his condition forbade his remaining there any longer.

The remedies hitherto prescribed had been given for mental symptoms, symptoms chosen somewhat at random, without regard to their due significance. A complete examination showed that Natrum sulphuricum was the indicated remedy. A thorough examination revealed an advanced leukaemia with probable tuberculosis of the bone marrow. A homoeopathic prescription, an immediate sojourn to the mountains and a suitable diet, transformed this young man in a few months. It was a careful diagnosis, therapeutic and nosologic, which enabled the physician to cure this youth.

6. A Boston physician told me of being called by a homoeopathic colleague to see a young man who had fallen backward upon a fence and suffered excruciating pains in the rectum. The pain had been somewhat relieved by doses of Arnica administered by a homoeopathic doctor. The patient had the sensation as if there was a splinter in the rectum. This symptom suggested to the doctor Nitric acid, then Hepar sulph, and then Silica. But the young man still suffered. After a few days of continued pain, the family insisted upon a consultation. The second homoeopathic doctor made an examination of the "site of pain", and found a splinter deeply embedded in the rectum. The extraction of this splinter and a careful diet for a few days, restored the patient.

   Here was an accident, not a sickness. Hence the physician should immediately make a pathological diagnosis and not prescribe disregarding a possible local cause. Had the mistake been made by a young practitioner, I should not comment upon it. But it occurred to a man who had been several years in general practice.

Source: June Vol LXVIII NO 810, 1933 Heal thyself

THERAPEUTIC AND PATHOLOGIC DIAGNOSIS THE PHYSICIAN'S RESPONSIBILITY

"Homoeopathic physician"—what meaning should this title convey?

The physician who, to the complete equipment of his university studies in medicine and surgery, adds also a thorough acquaintance with Homoeopathy and puts its principles into practice, only has the right to the title "homoeopathic physician". He will have made himself especially familiar with the work of Dr. Samuel HAHNEMANN, founder of Homoeopathy, with the **Materia Medica**, with the repertories and the laws related to the administration of remedies to the sick.

The study of Homoeopathy exacts of the neophyte a definite effort; for he must lay aside prejudices acquired during his university studies. But the method of considering any given case proves to be so different from that which he has hitherto known, that soon he sees the importance of this new method. Now he sees in the "cases" who come to consult him, not merely diseases which he must diagnose, but sick individuals, for whom he must find the similar remedy in his homoeopathic **Materia Medica**; a particular remedy for each, individually.

Also he must avoid routine; he may not remember other cases resembling this one, which he has already treated; he must isolate the distinctive difference in the sick person whom he now considers, must find out his peculiarities, his individual characteristics. This is a theory essentially and indispensably homoeopathic. Among the tangle of symptoms resulting from his examination, he must distinguish with care those which pertain to the sick one himself, as a thinking and suffering human being, because of which he is burdened with illness, from those others which concern only a portion of his physical organism - a single organ, or group of organs.

The practical result is fully inherent in this great secret of nature, discovered by Samuel HAHNEMANN: To determine the symptoms representative of the individual himself who is ill; and not make the blunder of noting alarming symptoms to any organ which is the point of least resistance where the illness finds for itself an exit, through which it utters its cry of pain.

A true homoeopath finds his task to consist first, in establishing a therapeutic diagnosis according to the fundamental laws of Homoeopathy discovered by

HAHNEMANN and developed by LIPPE, HERING, ALLEN, KENT, NASH and so many others.

This is which makes Homoeopathy a method not to be surpassed, this "therapeutic diagnosis", or I may call it "homoeopathic diagnosis", which leads to the remedy immediately without waiting for a "morbid diagnosis"; which treats a patient without having to determine his exact sickness! Observe that I say "exact sickness", for such general terms as hysteria, nervousness, rheumatism, dyscrasias or cryptogenic state, idiopathic, and what not - these do not deserve the noble term, "diagnosis". This fine and learned terminology readily covers the ignorance of the doctor giving treatment, an ignorance not as to his science but as to the case he deals with in a very different matter.

The word "diagnosis" alone connotes a pathological diagnosis, with verdict of morbidity. It is time to show to those who have not yet learned the fact, that there is a far more practical diagnosis: that is, one indicating from the very outset the necessary remedy. This is what Adolph LIPPE meant when he said: "Here is a person of the *Phosphorus* type: here, one of the *Arsenic* type; here, of *Pulsatilla*". And he uses the terms consecrated to these meanings by HAHNEMANN in the **Organon**, 1810. KENT also tells in his **Lectures on Homoeopathic Philosophy**, of a patient who asked him: "Doctor, what is the matter with me?" and he replied: "Why, you have *Nux vomica*," that being his remedy. Whereupon the old man said: "well, I did think I had some wonderful disease or other"! That is a therapeutic, a homoeopathic diagnosis.

I do not enlarge further upon the point; such diagnosis is clearly the first duty of the homoeopathic physician. Frequently it leads to a prompt, mild and permanent improvement, to a cure of the patient.

But we are not at the end of our task; we face two other heavy responsibilities: one of these concerns the patient, and the other, the future of medical science. Upon us rest both of these responsibilities.

As to the patient - our task is not only to relieve but to **Cure.** Now, a true cure rests not solely on a disappearance of existing symptoms, but equally on advice given the patient, that he need not again fall into such a state. Such counsels, of hygiene, of directing work and time, of morale, of reading, of the whole attitude and control of life - these also presuppose a diagnosis. And here, at this point, the nosological diagnosis becomes not only serviceable but indispensable to the doctor.(KENT's **Lectures on Homoeopathic Philosophy**, 1919, p. 143).

The whole idea of diagnosis, in relation to the task of the physician, is it not just the discovery of that famous **causa occasionalis** of which HAHNEMANN discussed in such detail? (See **Organon**, paragraphs 7, 73, 77, 150). The homoeopathic doctor must not simply prescribe pills or drops, but he must be a minister of nature, a "naturist", in addition to a homoeopathist, whose first purpose is, after securing the symptoms, to give them a diligent, interpretative analysis covering their last detail, a complete semeiologic examination.

There are homoeopaths, alas! who do not sufficiently examine even their patients, and who thus bring discredit upon the name and value of that medicine called homoeopathic. That certain clever men may omit such a procedure in examination as we have described, and still by a judicious interpretation of symptoms, cure their patient, is of course possible; but certainly such is not a method which could be generalized. Perhaps a few instances may clarify this thought yet further.

A young man of 18 years of age sought consultation regarding frequent attacks of angina, which settled as often on the right side as on the left, and followed almost regularly exposure to cold. Painting with various collutoria and frequent cauterizations and pulverisations in no way affected his condition and he asked my advice. The symptoms, as he gave them to me, pointed explicitly to *Tuberculinum* or *Sulphur*. Yet I gave neither of these remedies, because after further questioning I found that he wore low slippers and silk stockings, and that he took cold especially after dancing, or when his feet were cold. Accepting some simple hygienic advice, he wore thicker socks, shoes with rubber soles, gaiters in winter - and he had no more angina.

I acknowledge that possibly the remedy, had I given it, would have removed his tendency to the symptoms, in the bad conditions to which he exposed himself so often; but it seemed to me wiser to show him the mistake he was making, and to correct his state by simple hygienic measures. The therapeutic diagnosis was *Tuberculinum*; the morbid diagnosis was angina from exposure to cold; the prescription was hygienic advice. Result: a cure.

A young woman in domestic service, aged 20, came to consult me regarding rheumatism in the legs. She had been treated allopathically for three months, but the *salicylate* was making her deaf and producing vertigo. She found herself increasingly weak, walking with difficulty, vague pains and great weakness in the calves of her legs. Questioning led to a clear indication of *Lycopodium*, but I did not give that until completing the full examination. On reaching the throat, I found a curious condition of the pharynx; it looked as if painted with a yellow orange varnish. Taking a culture, I found a large number of Klebs-Loeffler bacilli, of the short type.

Evidently here there was paretic trouble sequelae of diphtheria, of which the angina had not been observed apart from a faint dryness of the throat, the sick girl had no other local symptoms. This diagnosis enabled me to isolate her and to take the measures necessary in this disease. Naturally, I made no serum, but for symptoms which I need not detail here, I gave one dose of *Lycopodium* 200, without observing any result in the following 15 days. The throat remained the same; weakness was still there; no improvement was perceptible. Such total failure of reaction to the indicated remedy led me to give her a dose *Diphtherinum* 200, to which the condition responded very well.

In ALLEN's **Nosodes** (1918, p.40) there is the following comment upon this remedy:

Painless diphtheria,

Symptoms almost entirely objective,

Patient too weak to complain, and apathetic

Prostration,

Highly susceptible to diphtheritic virus,

Post-diphtheritic paralysis

Remedy suitable when the most carefully selected remedy fails to relieve or permanently improve.

The girl's throat cleared up and resumed its normal aspect and at the end of a fortnight, another examination (made by the **Inst. Off. d'Hyg.**) showed not a single bacillus. Since the weakness remained, I gave then one dose of *Lycopodium*, of which the effect was surprising - the patient got up, began to walk, and in ten days was able to return to her position.

Would *Psorinum* or *Tuberculinum* have had an equally good effect? How could one determine the suitable nosode in a case which does not react save only by determining most carefully the exact nosological diagnosis?

A young man was treated by a homoeopath for submaxillary swelling. The homoeopathic treatment was changed frequently during several months, but without result. The doctor examined his neck each time, believing that here was a ganglionic condition. The patient consulted another physician who found in his face, head, and chest no remarkable signs; but on examining the spinal column, the physician found evidence of Pott's disease. The swelling was only a cold abscess arising from the third cervical vertebra. It was a tuberculosis of the bones of the spine, causing a suppuration which descending, went between the inter-aponeurotic spaces and settled in the submaxillary region.

The patient followed hygienic advice and suitable treatment until completely cured. Rest, mountain air, diet in accordance with the morbid diagnosis, a remedy based on the therapeutic diagnosis, made possible this desired result.

A patient, 55 years of age, was subject to colds in the head, was neurasthenic, and had suffered for six months from sudden attacks of suffocation. He had been treated by various allopathic physicians with all known anti-spasmodic and vagotonic medicines with no improvement whatever, but rather an increasing decrepitude. The patient walked with head bowed, had frequent loud eructations, spat continually, was afraid to swallow even his saliva. Eating was a veritable tragedy for him, for he remembered that his first attack had occurred while eating and he refused to take any liquid food, since this affected him more than solids. Finally, he gave up his doctors, for they but told him he was nervous, that he must make an effort to recover his health for himself, and that his attacks should be treated with contempt. A first examination revealed nothing obviously abnormal. For a time psychotherapy seemed to alleviate his fears. But neither *Mephitis, Ignatia* nor *Lachesis* could stop the attacks which though less frequent still did recur too often. But after taking cold, one time, laryngitis set in, causing a husky voice. However, remedies indicated had no effect. According to all homoeopathic principles the case was incurable. Examination of the larynx showed a paralysis of the right vocal cord; external examination revealed a thyroid tumor, very hard, and as large as a tangerine on the right side. This was the cause of the constriction of the recurrent nerve. His loss of weight, age, and complexion, and the development of symptoms, authorized the belief that here was a case of thyroid cancer, primary or metastatic it could not be determined. The prognosis was clearly not that of mere laryngitis. But the diagnosis indicated a very serious prognosis. Unfortunately the patient found Homoeopathy too slow, and returned to an allopathic physician, who applied radium needles to the tumor which reduced but ulcerated and within eight days, the poor patient died under terrible sufferings.

And again it is clear that the physician must know **what** he is treating quite as well as **whom** he is treating. What can be said of those who, not comprehending the case, called it "nerves", and ordered the sufferer to cure himself?

A young man of 20 had been treated for two years by a homoeopath with *Aurum, Calcarea, Ignatia, Pulsatilla*. He was in a neurasthenic state caused by frequent sudden attacks of vertigo which came upon him while working. He became so distressed, and depressed as actually to weep hot tears. He worked in a bank, but his condition forbade his remaining there any longer.

The remedies hitherto prescribed had been given for mental symptoms, symptoms chosen somewhat at random, without regard to their due significance—for mental symptoms have also their hierarchy, and must be known in their relationships. A complete examination showed that *Natrum sulphuricum*, was the indicated simillimum, thorough physical examination revealed an advanced myelogenic leukaemia with probable tuberculosis of the bone marrow. A homoeopathic prescription, an immediate sojourn in the mountains, with suitable diet, transformed this young man in a few months. Blood tests enabled me to follow the course of his steady gain and to control scientifically and objectively the course of subjective improvement as this followed.

But it was the two-fold diagnosis, therapeutic and nosologic, which enabled the physician to direct this unhappy youth toward the health from which he had so widely strayed.

A Boston physician told me of being called by a homoeopathic colleague in whose care was a young man injured by being impaled. He had fallen sitting upon a wooden paled fence and suffered excruciating pains in the rectum. The pain had been somewhat relieved by doses of homoeopathic *Arnica* administered by a homoeopathic doctor called in the emergency. The sensation as though there was a splinter in the rectum, suggested to the doctor *Nitric acid.*, *Hepar.*, then *Silicea*. But the young man still suffered. After a few days of continued pain, the family insisted upon a consultation. The second homoeopathic doctor, summoned, recalling section 7 of the Organon, made an examination of the "site of pain", and found indeed a splinter deeply imbedded in the rectum. The simple extraction of this splinter, and a diet for a few days, completely restored the patient. The wound closed without treatment.

Here evidently was an accident, not a sickness. Hence the physician should in such cases establish immediately the pathological diagnosis and not prescribe before he is sure whether there is a "local cause" or not. Had the mistake been made by a young practitioner, by a beginner, I should not comment upon it. But it was an occurrence in the experience of a man of long practice, over several years in general practice. And this seems to me to call for attention.

I beg that the ideas presented in this brief paper may be understood exactly as I intend them. Far be it from me to sermonize, or to give undue emphasis to nosological diagnosis. But it is indispensable that the conscientious physician be familiar with the interpretation of symptoms, with all that goes to insure a complete pathologic diagnosis, so that he shall not be in danger of making such blunders and oversights as those just cited.

Our responsibility demands that we establish a therapeutic diagnosis, but not less, a pathological one, as well. For the definition of a homoeopathic physician is, a physician who had **added** something special to his/her education. So that we must not, once entered upon practice, curtail this new special information, and neglect physical examinations. And it must be added that very often minute study of symptoms reported by the patient, will lead the doctor to conclude that there is a local cause which at first did not seem apparent. And the doctor must never forget to develop the essential quality: Good sense.

Nevertheless, whether in case of accident, or in case of illness, the distinction must be observed from the outset. As a homoeopathic physician he must make his therapeutic diagnosis; for if he prescribes for names of things, and not according to Hahnemannian rules he must be responsible for the failures that will result. Pathological diagnosis will claim his first attention in cases of accidents or indispositions.

We trust that in this study we have given each method its due place, insisting that we cannot omit either one or the other kind of diagnosis.

We always must have those two paragraphs of the **Organon** in mind (paragraphs 3 and 4):

The physician is likewise the guardian of health when he knows what are the objects that disturb it which produce and keep up disease and how to remove them from persons who are in health.

If the physician clearly perceives what is to be cured in disease, that is to say, in every individual case of disease (**knowledge of disease, indication**), if he clearly perceives what is curative in medicines, that is to say, in each individual medicine (**knowledge of medicinal powers**), and if he knows how to adapt, according to clearly defined principles, what is curative in medicines to what he has discovered to be undoubtedly morbid in the patient so that the recovery must ensue - to adapt it, as well in respect to the suitability of the medicine most appropriate according to its mode of action to the case before him (**choice of the remedy, the medicine indicated**) as also in respect to the exact mode of preparation and quantity of it required (**proper dose**) and the proper period for repeating the dose; if, finally, he knows the obstacles to recovery in each case and is aware how to remove them, so that the restoration may be permanent, then **he understands how to treat judiciously and rationally, then only can he merit the title genuine and true physician or a master in the art of healing.**

Source: The Homoeopathic Recorder, March 15, 1929

ON POTENCY CHOICE AND HOMOEOPATHIC POTENTISATION

First, a brief review regarding diagnosis which in Homoeopathy is two-fold:

I. The diagnosis of the **disease** according to the pathognomonic symptoms, with the help of general clinical status, through a specialist where necessary, through laboratory findings, X-rays, to clinch (a) what belongs to the exact disease, (b) what are conditioned by dietic and basic errors of hygiene, how defective are the home, clothing, care of the body, social life, regulation of life style, nutritional in-take etc.; also what could be set right without aid of medicament. Further to be considered are intoxications by alcohol, tobacco, narcotics, tranquilizers, sleeping drugs, drugs to calm down or excite etc. Such objective disease factors must be eliminated just as the physician of the old school does.

II. The diagnosis of the **sick person** to ascertain the non-pathognomonic symptoms which do not belong to the disease in question, the rare, strange, seldom, singular and which seem bizarre. These are symptoms which are contrary to common sense, make us reflect, and which are characteristic for a particular patient. Allopathy does not take into consideration such symptoms and considers the patient only as a hysteric or at the most handles such cases with suppressive remedies symptomatically which further add to the patient's sickness.

When the remedy to be given is chosen: which potency is to be prescribed?

This question can be settled only from practical experience. We must know that the HAHNEMANN-oriented physician employs basically **every** potency, from mother tincture to the highest potencies, M, 10M, CM, MM!

HAHNEMANN has, during his life time, fairly frequently varied the potency scale, just as the number of succussion strokes to be given in preparation of the potencies. He experimented, twice, ten times, hundred times, and more frequently to finally settle for ten strokes. He invented the centesimal potencies of C1 to C30 which he wrote as:0/VI that is 0 = globule and VI = sextillionth potency (= C18).

Regarding the preparation of this small dose HAHNEMANN has, in the **Organon**, paragraph 269, clarified the basic and essential difference between dilution, attenuation and potentisation. He wrote:

"It is heard every day that homoeopathic medicine potency is considered as mere attenuation, while it is the opposite of it, real development of the natural substance and bringing out the power lying concealed internally through friction and shaking, wherein a non-medicinal dilutant medium used is merely of secondary importance. Diluting alone, for example, dissolving a grain of salt it becomes mere water; the grain of salt disappears in theattenuation with plenty of water and will never by that become 'salt medicine' like our well prepared dynamisations raised to astonishingly high strength".

And as early as in 1886 the Geneva physician GRANIER wrote: "Production of a curative remedy from a substance is not reducing its powers but to develop the latent powers in it, potentising it, that is, to strip it of its material condition"

As I have already said, the potency choice is a question of practical experience. Indeed all homoeopaths have once begun with low potencies and have only tarried and without much conviction gone from the mother tincture up to C12. Others went up to C30 which for long remained the limit for HAHNEMANN and which he did not pass over.

What then is contained in a C30 which by the method of using of individual glass vials in which drops of the remedy in question are put and 99 drops of 90 percent alcohol is added and 10 strokes given repeatedly has acquired? And what are the high and highest potencies, the so-called Korsakoff potencies? The latter are prepared up to thousandth potency by the one glass method from the manually prepared C30, with 10 strokes by machine for every potency. Beyond the thousandth potency the **fluxion method** is used.

Everything regarding preparation of a homoeopathic medicine can be found in detail in the **Organon**. I recommend to you paragraph 123 as also paragraphs 264 to 272. With remarkable precision and conscientiousness HAHNEMANN has described there how the homoeopathic medicines must be prepared. Please study it thoroughly and attentively again.

Contrary to the general opinion KENT and his pupils were not in any way exclusively high potentists but they required all potencies from the mother tincture to the highest potencies. But their extensive experience and particularly their results made them give superior values to the high potencies because of their innumerable advantages.

Please bear in mind that the basis of the homoeopathic prescription is not the dose but it is the similie principle. This principle is of such a wonderful value that infact there is no limitation to the diminution of the concentration of the homoeopathic remedy if the actual symptoms of the patient harmonizes with the symptoms produced in the provings on the healthy.

Indeed the low potentists repeat the same objections as the allopaths do against the homoeopaths: how is it supposed to work when in the everyday diet and drinking water so many substances in weak doses are consumed?

I answer: It is not a question of academical dispute but is a matter of practical experience. What should one say about a case as follows? A splendid German shepherd-dog has been under the medical treatment of an eminent French veterinary physician for more than two months. The entire range of the most modern anti-infectious arsenals, Sulfonamide, the most effective antibiotics, for a sepsis with suppurative Metritis and Peritonitis have been used. On pressing the udder of the poor animal pus squirted out up to a litre in a day and that since weeks. This rotten pus stank disgustingly like rotten cheese. The dog was well looked after, cleaned every two hours and lied only in its owner's room. The mouth was completely dry, the weak animal could not move at all, refused food and was lying in a miserable state in the bed room. After 30 days of intensive treatment the veterinarian advised to give it an injection to put the animal to end since he had used the maximal doses of Sulphonamides etc., and felt that all that could be done had been done but failed and it was cruel to allow the animal to suffer further.

The owner of this dog who was my patient visited me one day for her monthly consultation and was in tears that she had to put an end to the life of the dog by agreeing to the injection.

I asked her: "but then why don't you allow it to be treated homoeopathically?" "But doctor, this is not the time for you to be witty. It is all right for me, since I have faith in it. But what would you do with your tiny pills to an animal which as the veterinarian says, is suffering from a Septicopyaemia?"

"Now madam, give the dog the medicine I will give you now and we will see later". I gave first *Staphylococcinum* 10M thrice a day. After two days *Pyrogenium* 10M. Two days later, because of the pus which was stinking like rotten cheese, *Hepar* 10M. Lastly after two more days because of the abundance of pus I gave *Medorrhinum* 10M. Now, from the very first dose the quantity of pus came down by 80%, the stink began to fade away slowly and after 8 days the dog was cured; it ran about, ate and slept just as when it was healthy.

In this of course all the potencies were prescribed in the ten thousandth! One can make fun of ten thousandth potencies and laugh. But how could a fatally ill condition like serious Septicaemia be got over and become normal and health restored? Materialistic homoeopaths will be easily confused in this. Behind this is nothing other than the grand law of similars discovered by HAHNEMANN. In paragraph 160 he says:

"As the homoeopathic medicine can never be made so small as to not be able to overcome it's analogous, non-long-standing, yet-unspoiled natural disease, could even thoroughly eradicate and cure, it can be understood as to why a dose which is not very smallest possible suitable homoeopathic medicine aroused always during the first hours after taking it, a perceptible homoeopathic aggravation".

And in paragraph 249a: "Since according to all experiences, almost no dose of a highly potentised specifically suitable homoeopathic medicine can be prepared which would be so small as not to bring about clear improvement in the disease for which it is suitable, so will it be injudicious and harmful to treat, if one were to repeat or increase the dose in the mistaken belief that its small aggravation or non-improvement, was because of its negligible quantity (it's far too small dose and it cannot therefore be of use)."

And in paragraph 279:

"These pure experiences point that ... the dose of the homoeopathically chosen highly potentised curative medicine for commencing treatment of a serious diseases (particularly chronic) can never as a rule be prepared so small as not be stronger than the natural disease, that it cannot, at least overcome a portion, eradicate at least a part of the sensations of the vital principle and thus cause commencement of the cure"

Ladies and Gentlemen, read these again and again and meditate on these observations of HAHNEMANN, strikingly corroborated here.

It is six months since that the dog became cured of a sepsis, a sepsis which materialistic allopathy with its "heroic" medicines could not treat, but on the contrary the condition became worse day by day and the veterinarian had given up all hopes.

How could it be argued against the allopath, the veterinarian and the low potentists?

I doubt much whether the C3 or C6 would have succeeded in a situation as this. Such a healing reveals four unquestionable facts:

1. Homoeopathy brings about cures when allopathy despite its modern toxic arsenals is powerless.

2. Homoeopathy, on the basis of the law of similars discovered by HAHNEMANN is able to make microbes and viruses, harmless.

3. The homoeopathic medicine in infinitesimal doses works qualitatively and not through its quantity.

4. Also that in an extremely serious, evidently fatal disease, the cure can be effected totally – "cito, tuto, et jecunde" as HAHNEMANN has impressed in the note to the first paragraph of his **Organon**.

I had a similar case of septicaemia from perforation of appendix and generalized peritonitis in a 10 year old child who had become parched and was lying in the Geneva Medical College Hospital awaiting his end after surgery. Neither the child nor the parents nor the Professor knew who had cured him. Only a single, really a single dose of *Arnica* 10M and then *Pyrogenium* 10M. I respect 10M.

To exclude every influence of direct or indirect suggestion, I have purposely chosen the case of an animal, so that the sceptics are convinced.

I will point out to you, that high potencies are of invaluable worth, that these small doses do not ever lose their therapeutic powers if they are protected from odours and had been prepared with due care. I own high potencies from HAHNEMANN's time, JENICHEN's for example. I have further such from the previous century as from FINCKE, SWAN, ALLEN, KENT which are still effective and dependable.

Innumerable physicians like NASH, KENT, CARLETON, Erastus CASE, GLADWIN, SHERWOOD, CUNNINGHAM, FINCKE, MAJUMDAR, Gibson MILLER, Mrs. TYLER, Sir John WEIR and others have published cures by high potencies.

HAHNEMANN, the founder of the homoeopathic principles had begun naturally from the mother tinctures, substantial medicines, materially and chemically analysable. Later he began to make the concentrations lesser by attenuations or triturations and observed that despite progressive division these substances remained more effective.

During his long life, ultimately he was 88 years old - HAHNEMANN was, in the opinion of his epoch, an exception, a revolutionary and in opposition to all practice and traditions. He went up to C30 wherein he used 30 separate 10 grams glass vials with 100 drops of alcohol in each. In the first vial he put one drop of the plant tincture or 5 grains of a chemical substance or the 3rd centesimal potency of an insoluble substance with which every passage was further attenuated in ratio of 1 to 100.

At the last stages of his life differences of opinion arose amongst his pupils. Some thought that underno circumstances should one go above the C30. Others among them his best pupil HERING and GROSS and others experimented with potencies upto 1000, 1500, 2000 and higher, saw with happy astonishment further successes. To avoid misunderstandings and hostilities from his pupils HAHNEMANN remained in the range of C30 although he had appreciated the efficiency of such high potencies.

Nevertheless, as researcher and experimenter he had recognized two interesting facts:

1. Some medicines possess, in specific potencies, an optimum efficiency in each case, whereof in the **Materia Medica Pura** HAHNEMANN indicated the third, sixth, twelfth and 30th as the most efficacious.

2. At the same time he observed that in general, the second, fourth and seventh potencies so to say, have a "shallow", decreased, reduced, curtailed efficacy - in short: a not excessively strong action is displayed, and that positive intervals between the individual potencies must be given. For this

reason his family medicine chest contained only the following potencies; 1- 3 - 6 - 9 - 12 - 24 and 30.

There was a time when FINCKE, ALLEN, SWAN and others were successful by employing highest potencies.

At a particular time there were high potentists, as they were called, who after the choice of the medicine according to symptom picture gave it in the highest available potency immediately at the beginning of the treatment. Dr A. NEBEL who practised here for quite long prescribed, for example, a CM or DM right at the first go, frequently with the best results, since the medicine chosen had been accurately specific.

KENT, a systematically experimenting mind endeavoured to find by innumerable experiments a rule or at least a scale method. After many trials over many years he set his scale method which I call the KENT scale. As KENT's pupils have since then corroborated, adherence to the following spacing gave the best results: 30, 200, 1M, 10M, 50M, CM, DM, MM.

KENT held, on the basis ofhis experience, the C30 as an excellent preparation to begin the treatment of a casesince it brought no, or hardly any, initial aggravation and with the 200th potency he considered them as low potencies with which, as already stated, treatment can be best commenced. He kept them particularly for the acute cases or chronic cases with objective and progressive organ changes. Otherwise he recommended in chronic cases the 1000th potency from which with appropriate time intervals which he could define after many years of experience, to go up to higher potencies.

After many years KENT could define the average duration of action of his high potencies. We have to respect these before repeating the dose. These are:

For 200: 3 to 4 weeks

M: at least 4 weeks

10M 5 weeks

50M 50 days

CM 3 months

DM 6 months

MM 1 year

Naturally these figures are to be considered as approximation, but all pupils of KENT have found these to be of superior practical value. Not in every case will it be suitable to repeat doses before expiry of this interval but only in combination with the other golden rule that no repetition before progressive amelioration ends.

The question of repetition of the dose, pharmacopollaxy as I would call it, was again modified by HAHNEMANN at the end of his life, in that he recommended continuous repetition of the dose daily despite favourable reaction. This method also I and many others have practised for a long time in the hope that it will render better and particularly speedier cures in chronic diseases. But soon because of the difficulties encountered by the patients regarding the taking too much or insufficiently, they attenuate it poorly and at will, repeat in irregular intervals, etc. - this method which is remarkable, is possible only in exceptional special cases which as I can vouch for, in actual practice is rarely seen. This reservation is so much more valid as through the KENT method also thoroughly remarkable successes can be obtained. Had HAHNEMANN known KENT who represented HAHNEMANN's continuance, he would have, without doubt, agreed with KENT's view, because it confirms absolutely to the essential principle of his teaching, "watch and wait", the careful observer's.

Today the knowledge that low potencies work better in acute, high in chronic cases, is more or less accepted by most of the homoeopaths. It all depends upon what one understands by low and high potencies.

The advantages of low potencies, including the C30 and 200 according to KENT is that it can be repeated without risk of severe aggravation. Why? Because a whooping cough, a diarrhoea with a frequent evacuation, tooth-aches, acute pains in general, the acute states so to say exhaust, consume, weaken the remedy so that in all cases where there is no reaction or where recurrence occurs such repetition is justified; for example in repeated vomiting repetition ofthe remedy once every two hours. It should be given after every vomiting.It can then be seen that the attacks become rarer until it passes off completely.

In chronic cases, the interval suggested by KENT, which has been verified, is to be followed.

The relapse of earlier symptoms, amelioration coming to a stand-still, status quo or the disease progressing further, are all indications for repetition of the dose.

Indeed it can be said that a master homoeopath is capable of results which the beginner is not able to. For example in some acute cases in which symptoms are painfully aggravated, like Sciatica, Otitis, Gastroenteritis, Acute Joint Rheumatism, a 10M produces a result which impresses by its rapid cure. It is like what WILLIAM TELL who with a single arrow directly pierced the apple on the head of his son.

I recommend to you, to first try C 30 and later go to the C 200. Now and again you can venture with a 10M if the indications for the medicine are clear and precise.

In coryza and minor colds *Aconitum napellus* 200 has at least 90% success. In certain chronic constipations immediate and sustained success from a single dose of *Nux vomica* 10M or *Bryonia* 10M is perceived.

I have cured the owner of a big restaurant who had been suffering for 14 years with a chronic constipation and who had been thoroughly stuffed with innumerable laxatives. There was nothing more which he had not tried. He had, however, further symptoms of *Nux vomica*, in his character, in his desires and aversions. A single dose of *Nux vomica* 10M has definitely cured him. Since then he has daily stool, "soft and gentile" as MOLIERE says, and he can have stools regularly with satisfaction.

A lady complained of headaches which localized in the occipital protuberance accompanied by constipation and eye pains which compelled her every 3 - 4 months to lie in a dark room since she could not bear the least light, and could not at all bear the sun. Every jolt, even walking aggravated. She also couldn't bend forward without the pain radiating to the neck. A single dose of *Bryonia alba* 10M at the close of an episode has put an end once for all her migraines which had been troubling her since 5 years for which she had taken a good quantity ofvarious medicaments.

These cases are not rare which you do not experience almost every day. When it happens: what happiness to the patients in the first place and also to the physician when he sees such conspicuous undeniable efficacy of the small doses which prove the value of the similie rule, the true basis of Homoeopathy.

Those who merely disparage and shake their heads have no idea about it and cannot gain the experience and observation. Of course, naturally the indications for the remedy prescribed must be exactly specific and symptomatology as defined by HAHNEMANN, KENT and their pupils, and not based otherwise on some one or the other. Because if the foundation is not based upon these propositions only failures will occur. If therefore Homoeopathy and high potencies are condemned it is not these but the prescriber himself who is at fault. Why is it that while others obtain successes it should be otherwise with him?

Study the **Materia Medica** thoroughly and diligently, study the **Organon** again and again and the philosophy of KENT. One of these days you will be compensated richly for that. Because Homoeopathy makes great demand of course but it compensates with high rewards. It is certain: Homoeopathy, practiced by earnest, persevering physicians with pleasure in their work, procures full satisfaction in material, intellectual and spiritual respects.

(Translated by Dr. K.S. Srinivasan, Madras).

THE DOSAGE USED BY HAHNEMANN

When from time to time at the Hahnemannian School the question of posology comes back for discussion, the Master's way is frequently mentioned by someone, but whatever is stated by one person is often contradicted by someone else; so that utter confusion reigns on the subject.

It occurred to me that this controversy could be finally settled if a chronological report was given based on the original documents of all of HAHNEMANN's writings on the question from his first publication until the end of his life.

I am well aware of the value of the material gathered by Dr. DUDGEON on the Hahnemannian posology in his **Lectures on Homoeopathy.** However, it is certain that, at that time, this esteemed authority lacked some very important information on the subject.

I am referring to HAHNEMANN's first edition of his **Materia Medica Pura**, of his "**Chronic Diseases**", and to the second edition of the first and second volumes of this work, as well as to the valuable compilation made by Dr. Richard HUGHESin 1878 which has been published in the British Journal of Homoeopathy. Through this source of information I was able to remedy certain lapses and make a complete expose of facts on the Hahnemannian posology from 1796 until HAHNEMANN's death in 1843. So here comes the sequence:

1796-1798: In 1796 HAHNEMANN stated for the first time, in the second volume of **"Hufeland's Journal"**, the homoeopathic doctrine in a paper entitled: **"Essay on a New Principle to Discover the Curative Virtues of Medicinal substances, Followed by Some Remarks on the Principles Accepted since Then."**

In this work he mentions several times the word "small doses", necessary when one prescribes drugs having similar action; but the context showed (and sometimes proved) that he thought the doses were so weak as to be unable to produce physiological effects with the substance used.

During the next two years it is clear that for the majority of the drugs used in his practice "small doses" never meant their use in fractionated parts. In 1797 he reported a case of colic for which he prescribed *Veratrum album* at a dose of 4 grains, i.e., 26 centigrams (1 grain = 0.065 centigrams) and a case of asthma treated with the same amount. In 1798 he reported a series of cases of fever, steady and remittent, which occurred that year and for which he prescribed *Arnica* (a few grains of the root, i.e. 15-30 centigrams.); *Ignatia*: for children seven to 12 years of age (2 to 3 grains, i.e. 12 to 18 centigrams); *Opium* (1/5 to 1/2 grain, i.e., 1 to 3 centigrams); *Camphora* (2 to 3 grains, i.e., 20 to 40 centigrams); *Ledum* (6 to 7 grains, i.e., 39 to 40 centigrams).

In another work published the same year, **"On a Few Periodical disease of the Daily Type,"** he mentions giving 8 grains, i.e., 52 centigrams, of *Ignatia* and doses of 1/2 to 1 drachm of *Cinchona* i.e., 2 to 4 grams of the raw substance.

So in the beginning HAHNEMANN used *substancial material doses*, corresponding approximately to those used in minimal doses by traditional medicine.

1799: This was the year of the sudden and unexplained introduction of what we now call "infinitesimal doses."In a publication "On the Care and Prevention of Scarlatina" (1801) HAHNEMANN mentions his treatment of an epidemic of this disease which occurred in the summer of 1799 and the use of our remedies: *Ipecac, Opium, Belladonna*, and *Chamomilla*, and speaks of each one prescribed in doses of a minuteness unknown in medical practice to that day.

His tincture of *Ipecacuanha*, for example, was made of one part of the drug to 2,000 parts of alcohol. Of this dilution only 1 to 10 drops were to be administered depending on the age of the patient.

Opium was diluted to such an extent that 1 drop was equivalent to 5 millionths of a grain (of about 6 centigrams). For children under four years of age this dose was to be further diluted to correspond to the 6X.

Belladonna was administered at a dose equivalent to the 432,000 part of a grain (i.e. 6 centigrams) of the extract, therefore approximately the 7th decimal dilution. As a prophylactic, a solution was prepared containing only 1/24 millionth part of a grain, of which 1 to 40 drops were prescribed depending on the age, and only every third day (i.e. about the 9th decimal dilution.)

Chamomilla tincture contained the 800th part of a grain of the dry extract, and only 1, 2 or more, drops were to be administered.

1801: In the second part of **"Hufeland's Journal"** for that year HAHNEMANN no longer needed to be defended on the question raised by his article: **"What could be the effects of such minute doses of *Belladonna*?"** But we should note that he mentions several times the effects of the millionth part of the ordinary dose, i.e. the 6th decimal or the 3rd centesimal:

"Those who are satisfied with these general indications will believe me when I state that I have cured various paralytic conditions by the administration for several weeks of a highly diluted solution of *Belladonna*. For the whole treatment I needed less than a 100 thousandth part of a grain of the extract, i.e. a 5th centesimal dilution or 10X. I also succeeded in curing several periodical nervous syndromes, furunculosis and its prevention, etc...with less than one millionth of a grain, i.e. a 6th CH for the whole treatment."

1806:HAHNEMANN says nothing more regarding the homeo posology, not even in his **Fragmenta de Viribus Medicamentorum Positivis** published in 1805, until his publication of **Medicine of Experience** in 1806 in **Hufeland's Journal**. Anyway, he does not go beyond the position he took in 1799 and even until 1801. He speaks of "the smallest possible sufficient dose," the exact number being of little importance; when referring to particular cases he mentions only 100th, 1,000th, one millionth of an ordinary dose, i.e., the 1st, 2nd, 3rd centesimal dilutions with which we are already familiar.

1809:I haven't been able to find anything regarding posology until 1809 aside from the general advice regarding the minuteness cited above.

In a study of more than 40 pages entitled: "**Reflections on the Three Methods Accredited for Treating Diseases**," published in Hufeland's Journal for that year, we find a paragraph stipulating that in certain circumstances of so-called "bilious states" one single unique dose of the tincture of *Arnica* root will suppress often within a few hours all fever, the bilious taste, and all the "intestinal storms."The tongue clears up and all vigor is restored before night.

However, in another communication published that year we note that regarding two violent poisons,

HAHNEMANN dilutes much more and much further than in the preceding three years.

For a fever that had lasted well over a year in Germany and described in the **"Allgemeine Anzeiger der Deutschen"** of 1809, he mentions *Nux vomica* and *Arsenicum*, according to the indicating symptoms, and recommends giving the first in the 3 millionth and the second in the 6 millionth of a grain, respectively in the 4th and 3rd centesimal dilutions.

1810:This is the historical year when the first edition of the **Organon** was published, and it is natural that we expect to find in the paragraphs devoted to posology a whole series of extra details regarding the homoeo dilutions. However, there is very little else said aside from what was reported in his **Medicine of Experience** of 1805.

In a note which I have been able to trace in the **Organon** paragraph 247 HAHNEMANN writes (according to R. HUGHES): "When I speak of the dose prescribed in homeo practice as being the smallest possible, I do not intend - because of the difference in pharmacological power - to give a precise table of the volume and weights of each drug."

1814: in an article on the **"Treatment of Typhus and the Nervous Hospital Fever spreading Now."** (it was the time of Germany's insurrection against Napoleon following his retreat from Russia) in 1814 we have a new glimpse of HAHNEMANN's Posology.

The drugs he recommended, according to the symptomatology, were *Bryonia, Rhus-tox,* and *Hyoscyamus.* He suggested the administration of the first two in the 12th dilution, the third in the 8th dilution, however on a different scale of the centesimal, which was his usual practice and in which 6 drachms, i.e., 1,000 drops instead of 100 drops of alcohol, had to be used in each progression of the dynamisation.

This would correspond, according to Dr. DUDGEON, to the 12th dilution being equivalent to our 15th to 16th dilution; and the 8th, to our 10th approximately.

Spiritus nitri dulcis was indicated in certain circumstances, and 1 drop had to be successed in 30 cc. of water and the mixture consumed in 24 hours.

1816: This year is outstanding in the history of Hahnemannian posology, at least from my knowledge of books.

In the first volume of **Materia Medica Pura**, published in 1811, HAHNEMANN fails to give any details in his preliminary remarks to the many pathogeneses regarding the dose of the drugs he found to be particularly indicated.

We know nothing of his views at that time regarding the dosage of *Belladonna, Dulcamara, Cina, Cannabis, Cocculus, Nux vomica, Opium, Moschus, Oleander, Mercurius, Aconite* and *Arnica.*

Now, however, in the second volume, published in 1816, and in the next two, the best dose of each drug is indicated.

For *Causticum*, for example, 1 drop of the original preparation corresponds to one dose.

Arsenicum is to be administered at the 12th, 18th, or at the 30th dilution, and preferably the 30th.

For *Ferrum* the 100th, the 10,000th, and the 50,000th part of a grain is advised as the best dose.

Ignatia is recommended at the 9th or at the 12th dynamisation, and *Rheum*, in acute cases, at the 9th.

For *Pulsatilla, Rhus-tox,* and *Bryonia* the same doses are indicated:

If the patient is robust and his disease is of some duration, 1 drop of the pure juice of the plant is the best dose. But in delicate patients and for acute conditions the dose is to be smaller: for *Pulsatilla*, the 12th; for *Rhus-tox*, the 12th or the 15th dilution; and for*Bryonia*, the 18th dilution.

These ideas are perfectly illustrated in two famous cases published at that time by HAHNEMANN as examples of homoetherapeutics, as cited in the preface of that volume.

The first case involved a gastralgia with gastrosuccorrhoea of three weeks' duration in a robust woman with otherwise good health.

As predicted by HAHNEMANN, she was cured in less than 24 hours by a single drop of the root of *Bryonia*, as verified by one of his friends.

The second case was an acute gastritis of five days' duration in a pale and weak man of 42 years of age. His remedy was 1/2 drop of the 12th dilution of *Pulsatilla*. The next day good digestion was restored, and a week later, when HAHNEMANN checked him, the cure was well maintained.

These two cases were treated at the end of 1815.

Furthermore, HAHNEMANN was then 60 years of age. In the same preface we learn that he had now adopted the centesimal scale, the greatest care to be taken so that each dynamization would be exactly what it was supposed to be; but, alas, the pharmacists failed to follow his instructions.

The dried plants are to be treated with 20 parts of alcohol. Each drop of that mother tincture is estimated as containing 1/20th part of the medicinal power (Arzneikraft) of that preparation. The tinctures prepared with fresh plants by mixing the expressed juice with equal parts of alcohol, are to be considered as titrated at 50 %. Therefore 2 drops will be added to 98 drops of alcohol to obtain the 1st centesimal dilution.

(Translated by Roger A. SCHMIDT, M.D. from Groupement Hahnemannian de Lyon, 9th series, No.1, 1972, p.35-41).

SOURCE OF THE ARTICLES

1. THE HAHNEMANNIAN GLEANINGS, VOL. XLVI, JAN. 1979.

2. THE HAHNEMANNIAN GLEANINGS, VOL. XIVI, AUG. 1979.

3. THE HAHNEMANNIAN GLEANINGS, VOL. XLVII, APR. 1980.

4. THE HAHNEMANNIAN GLEANINGS, VOL. XXXIX, MARCH 1972.

5. THE HOMOEOPATHIC RECORDER, NOV. 1929, CURRENT HOMOEOPATHIC PERIODICALS

6. THE HAHNEMANNIAN GLEANINGS, VOL. XL, APRIL 1973.

7. THE HAHNEMANNIAN GLEANINGS, VOL. XLI, MARCH 1974

8. THE HAHNEMANNIAN GLEANINGS, VOL. XLIV, DEC. 1977.

9. ZEITSCHRIFT FÜR KLASSISCHE HOMÖOPATHIE, 2, 1964.

10. THE HAHNEMANNIAN GLEANINGS, VOL. XLIV, JAN, 1977.

11. THE HOMOEOPATHIC HERITAGE, VOL. III, APRIL AND MAY 1978.

12. THE HOMOEOPATHIC HERITAGE, VOL. III, FEBRUARY 1978.

13. ZEITSCHRIFT FÜR KLASSISCHE HOMÖOPATHIE, BAND 29, 1985.

14. THE HOMOEOPATHIC HERITAGE, JAN. 1978.

15. JOURNAL OF AMERICAN INSTITUTE HOMOEOPATHY, JUNE 1974.

[1] When they were not caused by an important error in regimen, a violent emotion, or a tumultuous revolution in the organism, such as the occurrence or cessation of the menses, conception, childbirth and so forth."

[2] "In cases where the patient (which, rarely happens in chronic, but not infrequently in acute diseases) feels very ill, although his symptoms are very distinct, so that this state may be attributed more to the benumbed state of the nerve, which does not permit the patient's pains and sufferings to be distinctly perceived, this torpor of the internal sensibility is removed by *Opium*, and in its secondary action the symptoms of the disease become distinctly apparent".

[3] See page 84.

[4] "One of the many great and pernicious blunders of the old school."

[5] In the Introduction to the **Organon I** (1810) HAHNEMANN says, "..... In this investigation I found the way to the truth, but I had to tread it alone......the farther I advanced from truth to truth......" in a Note dated 12th March 1843 HAHNEMANN wrote "I sought truth earnestly and found it." = KSS.

[6] Kent: Lectures on Homoeopathic Philosophy; Lecture V

[7] Poincaré, H.: La Valeur de la Science.

[8] Larousse: Encyclopaedia

[9] Regnualt: Precis de logique evolutionniste. Bib.phil. p.118.

[10] Boutroux: Loc.cit.

[11] Littré. Dictionary of Medicine, Art: Law.

[12] It is also very useful in fractures when small bone chips remain in the wound. The *Silica* patient is always very chilly, mostly in the head, and shows frequent little white spots on the nails, called 'flores unguis' or leukonychia striata. (Repertory p.1191, Extremities, spotted nails.)

A DAYS WORK

[Dr. Schmidts article will be of particular interest to readers because he is one of the leading high potency men. He uses almost exclusively high and the very highest potencies in very infrequent doses, following the examples of Dr. Samuel Hahnemann, whose favourite potency was the 30th.—J.E.B.].

I WOULD warn the readers of this article not to jump to the conclusion that the remedy which I have successfully employed for some disease or other can safely be used in the hope of success in every case of the same disease. Diseases should be treated not in accordance with their names, but in accordance with the totality of symptoms of the patient. In giving the briefest summary of days work, I wish merely to show the all- sufficiency of the homoeopathic law and the fact that interesting and valuable results may be obtained by acting in accordance with that law. I would mention that Hahnemann published only a very few cures of his own because he wished to prevent his followers from acting mechanically and prescribing for the names of diseases instead of for the totality of symptoms, irrespective of the official designation of the complaint treated.

ACUTE COLIC ORIGINATING IN THE LIVER—Cured by three doses of Belladonna 200th potency in a few hours.

WHITLOW OF THE FINGER.—Very painful, was treated with a dose of Anthracinum 200th potency, and then with Hepar sulphuris 1000th, and is rapidly getting well.

ASTHMA.—A clergyman who had suffered for several years from this disease was rapidly improved with Natrum sulphuricum in doses which were gradually raised from the 1,000th potency to 500,000th potency.

ANAEMIA OF PRE-TUBERCULOUS CHARACTER.—A young girl, who suffered from this complaint, combined with very painful menstruation, was greatly relieved with Pulsatilla in the 10,000th potency.

APOPLEXY.—A man of 50 had had two apoplectic strokes followed by complete paralysis of the left side. His condition was greatly improved and he was enabled to walk almost normally and to speak, with a few doses of Phosphorus, one in the 1,000th potency, followed by a dose in the 10,000th potency and one in the 50,000th potency with an interval of from five to seven weeks between each dose. During eleven months there has been no relapse. There were two crises which occurred with an interval of three weeks.

ST. VITUS DANCE.—This disease in a backward girl of 15 years who had not yet menstruated and had a very thick neck, was greatly improved with the help of Agaricus followed by Cuprum and then by Calcarea silicata, all in high dilutions.

PERIODIC HEADACHES.—A lady of 45 with this trouble is doing well with Nux vomica 10,000th and higher.

ECZEMA ALL OVER THE BODY AND ACUTE ARTHRITIS.—A lady in this condition, 44 years old, is doing well, having received a dose of Arsenic in the 1,000th potency, and another dose in the 50,000th potency.

INFLAMMATION OF THE TESTICLES.—This trouble, combined with varicocele and neurasthenia, in the case of a young man of 20 was wonderfully improved in less than a month after two years sufferings from these complaints. He was given Arsenicum in the 1,000th potency.

SPASMS OF THE OESOPHAGUS.—A youth of 12 suffered from spasms of the swallowing tube, which caused him to vomit his food. His condition was greatly improved by a dose of Sulphur in the 1,000th potency, followed by Lachesis in the 10,000th potency.

MIND AFFECTION AT THE CHANGE OF LIFE.—A lady, 40 years old, suddenly had the sensation that she was living in a different world. Everything around her seemed strange to her, she knew no longer where she was and she suffered mental agonies in consequence.

She was cured in a few months with Medorrhinum given consecutively in the 1,000th, the 10,000th and 50,000th potency.

TUMOUR OF THE BREAST.—A lady of 38 was cured of a breast tumour with Silica, but other tumours appeared afterwards in the other breast.

ASTHMA.—A lady, 42 years old, had been suffering for eight years from asthma. She was cured in a month with a dose of Arsenic in the 1,000th potency, followed by Arsenic in the 10,000th potency, and the cure has remained for two years.

ASTHMA.—A girl of 15 with asthma is at present being treated and her condition has been greatly improved with Syphilinum 200th potency.

SYRINGOMYELIA.—A young man, suffering from this disease of the spinal cord was wonderfully improved and nearly cured in the course of six months with Phosphorus in the 1,000th and the 10,000th potency.

HAEMORRHAGE AND FIBROID TUMOUR AT THE CHANCE OF LIFE.—The haemorrhage and all other disagreeable symptoms were cured in the course of a year with Lachesis, followed by Phosphorus, both given in high potencies.

NERVOUS BREAKDOWN.—A young girl, who suffered from neurasthenia owing to sorrow caused by a love affair, was cured in three weeks with Ignatia in the 10,000th.

NERVOUS FEARS.—A lady of 54, who suffered because she feared to meet people, to go into crowds, and to go out because she dreaded that she would not be able to find a public convenience, was cured in six months with Sulphur in the 1,000th potency.

SWALLOWING TROUBLE.—A child of 2 was brought to me and the mother told me that it was unable to swallow any solid food. It could not masticate and would take no nourishment except liquids. The child suffered also from facial eczema which had been in existence for several months. A single dose of Calcarea in the 1,000th potency enable the mother, to her great surprise, to feed the child on solid food, biscuits, etc. The child rapidly learned to masticate thoroughly and within six weeks the eczema had completely disappeared.

These few cases are come of the patients whom I have seen in the course of a day. They gladden the heart of a homoeopath, for they show the efficacy of the law of similars by his cures with highly potentized medicines. Ones satisfaction to produce cures like those described is increased by their having been brought about by a single remedy which was allowed to develop its full power of action before another dose of the same medicine in the same or in a higher potency was prescribed. Besides, no change of medicine was undertaken until the effect of the dose originally given had become fully established. If one changes haphazard from one medicine to the other or prescribes several medicines at the same time, one knows no longer which medicine has been responsible for improvement or for a cure.

Source: Oct. LXVIII No 814, 1933 Heal thyself.

REMEDIES AGAINST THE THREE CHRONIC MIASMS OF HAHNEMANN (PSORA, SYCOSIS, SYPHILIS)

A list of Antipsorics, Ant syphilitics and Anti sycotics is appended. The better and correct designations would be "Homoeopsorics", "Homoeosyphilitics" and "Homoeosycotics" because the Homoeology requires differentiation of the following three designations:

The word Antidote should be banished from our vocabulary. The root "anti" comes either from the Latin "ante" or the Greek "anti". The Latin word "ante" indicates an occurence, temporal and spatial, for example; antedating, antechamber, anticipation, etc. Often it is presented radically in the Latin form "ante" as for example by the expressions: antediluvian, antecedents, etc.

The Greek root "anti", on the other hand, indicates "against", opposition: antidote, antisyphilitic, antipsoric, etc. GRANIER (Homoeolexique) opines that, if we mean the Greek root then the word does not fit into our (homoeopathic) vocabulary because, it should be "Homoeo" in our case, and in no case "anti". Dr. ROUX, a Frenchman, has already pointed out to us that it was absurd for us to speak of "antipsorics" etc. He is the first who suggested the expressions "Homoeopsoric", "Homoeosyphilitic", "Homoeosycotic".

GALEN considered all internally administered medicines as "antidotes". The old school (Allopathy) employed the term Antidote as Synonym for the opposing toxin. When we speak of antidote we imagine an opposite toxin. So in the old school. The medicine used for example in a case of poisoning is not basically a "contra" but a "pro" and instead of antidote we would better say 'Prodote'.

When we want to remove with our medicine the effects of a wrong medicine or a too energetic medicine or would like to diminish its effects then the proper designation for that medicine would be Diadot; whereas the term Homoeodot is closer to the dynamic action of our medicines because we are neutralising a disease cause or a dynamised medicine with another similarly dynamised substance according to the law of similars.

I have taken the trouble of collecting from our literature an exact List of the Homoeopsorics, Homoeosyphilitics and Homoeosycotics. Among the authors consulted HAHNEMANN, the founder of this concept comes first. Then BOENNINGHAUSEN's great work on what he called as Antipsorics and further HARTLAUB and TRINKS, KENT, GIBSON-MILLER, PETROZ etc. Evidently I have taken all the remedies from HAHNEMANN's **Chronic Diseases** which are all found in KENT's Repertory. Only in CLARKE's I found *Thyroidinum* mentioned as Homoeosyphilitic.

HOMOEOPSORICA

Aconitum napellus A. T.

Aesculus hippocastanumA.

Agaricus muscarius H. B. A. G.

Alumina (argile) H. B. A. G.

Ambra grisea A. T. B. Gr.

Ammonium carbonicum H. T. B. A. G.

Ammonium muriaticum H. B. A. G.

Amygdalus amara T. B.

Anacardium orientale H. T. B. A. G.

Angustura vera T.

Antimonium crudum H. T. B. A.

Antimonium tartaricum T. B. A.

Apis mellifica H. G.

Argentum metallicum H. A. G.

Argentum nitricum T. B. Gr.

Arnica montana T.B.

Arsenicum album H.T.B.A.G.

Arsenicum jodatum A.

Asafoetida T.B.S.

Asarum europaeum T.B.

Aurum foliatum H.T.B.G.

Aurum muriaticum B.

Baryta acetica T.B.

Baryta carbonica H.T.B.G.

Belladonna atropa H.T.B.A. Gr. Ae

Berberis vulgaris A.

Bismuthum nitricum T.B.

Boracis acidum H.

Bovista lycoperdon B.A.

Bryonia alba T.B. Ae

Bufo ranaA.

Calcarea acetica B.

Calcarea ostrearum H.T.B.G.

Calcarea phosphorica H.A.G.

Calcarea sulfurica T.B.

Camphora officinalis T.B.

Cannabis sativa T.B.

Cantharis vesicatoria T.B.

Capsicum annum T.B

Carbo animalis H.T.B.G..

Carbo vegetabilis H.T.B.G..

Causticum H.T.B.G.Cl.

Chamomilla matricaria T.B.

Chelidonium majus T.B.

China officinalis T.A.

Cicuta virosa T.B.A.

Cina semen contra T.B.

Cinnabaris A.

Clematis erecta H.T.B.G.S. Gr.

Coca erythroxylon A.

Cocculus indicus T.B.A.

Coffea cruda T.A.

Colchicum autumnale T.B.

Colocynthis cucumis H.T.B.A.

Conium maculatum H.T.B.G

Crocus sativus T.B.A.

Cuprum metallicum H.T.B.A.G.S. Gr.

Cyclamen europaeum T.B. Gr.

Daphne indica

Digitalis purpurea H.T.B.

Drosera rotundifolia T. Ae.

Dulcamara solanum H.T.B.G.

Electricitas positiva T.

Euphorbium cyparissias T

Euphorbium dulcis T.

Euphorbium dulcis T.

Euphorbium lathyris T.

Euphorbium officinarum H.B.G. Gr.

Euphrasia officinalis Gr.

Ferrum magneticum T.

Ferrum metallicum B.A.G.S. Gr.

Ferrum phosphoricum K.

Flouris acidum A.G.

Galvanismus T.

Graphites mineralis H.T.B.A.G.

Guajacum officinale H.T.B.G.

Hamameliss virginica A.

Helleborus niger T.

Helonias diocia A.

Hepar sulfuris calcareum H.B.G.S. Gr.

Hydrasris canadensis G.

Hydrocyanic acidum T.

Hyoscyamus niger T.A.

Ignatia amara T.A.

Iodum H.T.B.A.G.

Ipecacuanha cephaëlis T.A.

Kalium bichromicumG.

Kalium carbonicum H.B.A.G.

Kalium iodatum B.A.G. Gr. K

Kalium nitricum H.B.G.

Kalium phosphoricum K.

Lac caninum A.

Lac defloratum A.

Lachesis trigonocephalus G.

Laurocerasus prunus T.

Ledum palustre T.

Lilium tigrinum A.

Lobelia inflata A.

Lycopodium clavatum H.T.B.G.

Magnesia carbonica H.T.B.A.G.

Magnesia muriatica H.T.B.G.

Magnetis polus arcticus T.

Magnetis polus australis T.

Manganum aceticum H.T.B.G.

Mercurius corrosivus T.

Mercurius solubilis T.A.K.

Mezereum daphne H.T.B.G.

Millefolium achillea A.

Morphinum

Moschus moschiferus T.

Murex purpurea A.

Muriatis acidum H.T.B.A.G.

Natrium carbonicum H.T.B.A.G.

Natrium muriaticum H.B.A.G.

Niccolum metallicum B.S.Gr.

Nitri acidum H.T.B.G.

Nux vomica T.A.

Oleander nerium T.

Oleum hecoris aselli A.

Opium somniferum T.

Origanum majorana A.

Paris quadrifolia T.

Petroleum H.T.B.A.G

Phosphori acidum H.T.B.G.

Phosphorus H.T.B.A.G.

Platina H.T.B.A.G.S.Gr.

Plumbum aceticum T.Gr.

Plumbum metallicum B.G.S.

Plumbum muriaticum T.

Podophylum peltatumK.

Psorinum A.G.

Pulsatilla nigricans T.A.

Rananculus bulbosus A.S. Gr. Ae.

Rheum officinale T.

Rhododendron chrysanthum H.B. Gr.

Rhus toxicodendron T.B.S. Gr. Ae.

Rumex crispus G.

Ruta graveolens T.G.

Sabadilla officinarum T.B.

Sabina juniperus T.K.

Sambucus nigra T.

Sarracenia purpurea A.

Sarsaparilla smilax H.T.B.G.K.

Scilla maritima T.

Secale cornutum A.K.

Selenium B.S.

Senega polygala H.B.

Silicea H.T.B.A.G.

Spigelia anthelmia T.B.S. Gr.

Spongia tosta T.G. Gr.

Stannum metallicum H.T.B.A.G

Staphysagria delphinum B.A.S.Gr.K.

Stramonium datura T.

Strontiana carbonica B.

Sulfur iotum H.T.B.A.G

Sulfuris acidum H.B.G.

Taraxacum dens leonis T.

Teucrium marum verum T.

Thuja occidentalis T. Ae.

Trifolium pratense T.

Tuberculinum bovinum K.

Veratrum album T.

Zincum metallicum H.T.B.A.G.K.

HOMÖSYCOTICA

Aesculus hippocastanum A.

Agaricus muscarius A.K.

Alumen K.

Alumina A.K.

Ammonium carbonicum A.K.

Ammonium muriaticum A.

Anacardium orientale H.A.G.K.

Anatherum muricatum A.

Angustura vera A.

Antimonium crudum H.A.G.K.

Antimonium tartaricum H.G.K.

Apis mellifica H.A.G.K.

Aranea diadema H.G.K.

ARGENTUM METALLICUM H.A.G.K.

ARGENTUM NITRICUM A.K.

Armoracia A.

Arsenicum album B.A.

Asa foetida A.

Asarum europaeum A.

Asparagus A.

Asterias rubens G.K.

Aurum foliatumG.K.

Aurum muriaticum G.K.

Baryta carbonica A.G.K.

Benzoicum acidum A.

Berberis vulgaris A.

Borax veneta A.K.

Bovista lycoperdon A.

Bryonia alba A.G.K.

Bufo rana A.

Caladium seguinum A.

Calcarea ostrearum A.K.

Cannabis indica A.

Cannabis sativa A.

Cantharis vesicatoria A.

Capsicum annuum A.

Carbo animalis G.K.

Carbo vegetabilis A.G.K.

Carbolic acidum A.

Carboneum sulfuratum K.

Caulophylum thalictroides A.

Causticum A.G.Cl.K.

Cedron simaruba A.

Chamomilla matricaria A.L.G.K.

Chimaphila umbellata A.

China officinalis

Cicuta virosa A.

Cimicifuga A.

Cinnabaris L.G.

Clematis erecta A.K.

Coccus cacti A.

Colchicum autumnale A.

Colocynthis cucumis A.

Conium maculatum A.G.K.

Copaiva officinalis A.

Crocus sativus A.

Crotalus horridus A.

Croton tiglium A.

Cubeba officinalis A.

Cuprum aceticum

Cyclamen europaeum A.

Digitalis purpurea A.

Doryphora decemlineata A.

Dulcamara solanum A.G.K.

Epigaea repens A.

Erechthites hieracifolia A.

Erigeron canadense A.

Eupatorim purpureum A.

Euphorbium purpureum A.

Euphorbia pilulifera A.

Euphorbium officinarum L.

Euphrasia officinalis A.G.K.

Fagopyrum esculentum A.

Ferrum metallicum G.K.

Fluoris acidum A.G.K.

Gambogia (Gummi gutti) A.

Gelsemium sempervirens A.

Gnaphalium polycephalum A.

Graphites G.K.

Helonias diocia A.

Hepar sulfuris calcarea G.K.

Hydrastis canadensis A.

Influenzinum A.

Iodum G.K.

Kalium bichromicum A.

Kalium carbonicum A.G.K.

Kalium iodatum A.

Kalium muriaticum A.

Kalium nitricum A.

KALIUM SULFURICUM A. K.

Kalmia latifolia G.

Lac caninum A.

Lachesis trigonocephalus A.G.K.

Lilium tigrinum A.

Lithium carbonicum A.

Lycopodium clavatum A.L.G.K.

Magnesia carbonica A.

Manganum aceticum A.K.

MEDORRHINUM A.K.

Mercurius dulcis A.

Mercurius solubilis A.G.K.

Mezereum daphne A.G.K.

Moschus moschiferus A.

Murex purpurea A.

Natrium carbonicum A.

Natrium muriaticum A.

NATRIUM SULFURICUM A.K.

NITRIC ACIDUM L.A.K.

Nux vomicaL.(A).

Oleum jecoris aselli A.

Origanum vulgare

Palladium A.

Papaya vulgaris A.

Pareira brava A.

Petroleum G.K.

Petroselinum sativum A.

Phosphoric acidum L.

Phosphorus L.

Phytolacca decandra A.G.K.

Piper nigrum A.

Platina

Plumbum

Prunus spinosa A.

Psorinum L.

Pulsatilla nigricans A.K.

Ratanhiaaa peruviana A.

Rhus toxicodendron A.

Sabadilla officinarum

Sabina juniperus L.A.K.

Saccharum lactis A.

Sanicula aqua A.

Sarracenia purpurea A.

Sarsaparilla smilax A.G.K.

Secale cornutum A.G.K.

Selenium G.K.

Senecio aureus A.

Senega polygala A.

SEPIA SUCCUS A.K.

Silicea A.G.K.

Spigelia anthelmica B.

STAPHYSAGRIA DELPHINUM L.A.K.

Stillingia silvatica A.

Stramonium datura A.

Sulphur iotum A.G.K.

Tabacum nicotiana A.

Terebinthinae oleum A.

THUJA OCCIDENTALIS B.L.A.K.

Uranium nitricum A.

Viburnum opulus A.

HOMÖOSYPHILITICA

Argentum metallicum K.

Arsenicum album A.G.K.

ARSENICUM IODATUM A.K.

Arsenicum sulfuratum flavum K.

Asafoetida L.A.G.K.

AURUM FOLIATUM L.K.

AURUM MURIATICUM G.K.

AURUM MURIATICUM NATRONATUM K.

Badiaga fluviatilis G.K.

Belladonna atropa A.

Benzoic acidum G.K.

Calcarea iodata K.

Calcarea sulfurica K.

Carbo animalis G.K.

Carbo vegetabilis G.K.

Causticum Cl.

Cinnabaris A.G.K.

Clematis erecta K.

Conium maculatum K.

Corallium rubrumG.K.

Crotallus horridus G.K.

Ferrrum metallicum A.

Flouris acidum L.A.G.K.

Guaicum officinale K.

Hepar sulphuris calcareum L.G.K.

Iacaranda caroba A.K.

Iodum L.

Kalium arsenicosum K.

Kalium bichromicum L.G.K.

Kalium carbonicum A.

Kalium chloratum K.

KALIUM IODATUM A.K.

KALIUM SULFURICUM G.K.

Kalmia latifolia

Lac caninum L.G.

Lac defloratum A.

Lachesis trigonocephalus G.K.

Ledum palustre K.

Lycopodium clavatum G.K.

MERCURIUS B.L.A.K.

MERCURIUS CORROSIVUS K.

Mercurius dulcis A.

MERCURIUS IODATUS FLAVUS G.K.

MERCURIUS IODATUS RUBER G.K.

Mercurius vivus B.

Mezereum daphne L.A.G.K.

Millefolium achillea A.

NITRIC ACIDUM L.A.K.

PetroleumG.K.

Phosphoric acidum G.K.

Phosphorus G.K.

PHYTOLACCA DECANDRA L.K.

Sarsaparilla smilax L.A.G.K.

Secale cornutum A.K.

SILICEA A.G.K.

Staphysagria delphinum A.G.K.

STILLINGIA SILVATIC AG.K.

Sulphur iodatum K.

Sulphur iotum G.K.

SYPHILINUM A.K.

Thuja occidentalis G.K.

Thyroidinum Cl.

LITERATURE

(H.) - HAHNEMANN S: Die Chronischen Krankheitan, 4 Bände. Dresden und Leipzig 1835.

(T) - HARTLAUB & TRINKS: Systematische Darstellung der antipsorischen

Arzneimittel in ihren reinen Wirkungen. 3. Bd., S.203. Dresden 1830

(B.) - von BOENNINGHAUSEN C.: Repertoriumder-homoopathischen Arzneien, 2 Bände, Munster 1832,1833,1835.

(L.) - LIPPE C.: Repertory to the more charasteric symptoms of the Materica medica, lere ed. 1879-2e ed. 1881

(A.) - ALLEN J.H.: The Chronic Miasms,2 vol. 1990

(G.) - MILLER Gibson: Journal of Homoeopathics-supplt.-oct.1990

(Cl.) - CLARKE: Dictionary of practical **Materia Medica**. London 1990

(S.) - STAPF}

(Gr.) - GROSS}—zit. Nach v. BOENNINGHAUSEN.

(Ae.) - AEGIDI}

(P.)- PETROZ

(K.) - KENT J. T.: Repertory of the **Materia Medica**, 6e ed. 1957-**Materia Medica**, 2e ed. 1911

- HAEHL R.: Samuel Hahnemann-Sein Leben und Schaffen, Bd. II, S.163. LEIPZIG 1922